Poverty

Poverty is one of the longest-standing problems facing governments and populations throughout the world. Whether in prosperous times or during depressions, whether in agricultural, industrial or post-industrial societies, no matter how it is measured and despite anti-poverty programmes and aid to the poor, poverty continues. The poverty rate in the industrialised West ranges between 10 and 15 per cent and is much higher in agricultural societies. In post-socialist countries it is only beginning to be admitted and identified.

The chapters of *Poverty* focus on ten different countries (USA, UK, Australia, Canada, Hong Kong, Ireland, Malta, the Netherlands, Philippines and Zimbabwe) and the socio-economic and historical context within which poverty exists, the extent and nature of poverty, the causes of poverty, and measures that have been taken to mitigate poverty.

John Dixon is a Senior Lecturer in the Department of Social Policy and Social Work, University of Plymouth. **David Macarov** is an Emeritus Professor in the Paul Baerwald School of Social Work, The Hebrew University, Jerusalem.

Poverty

A persistent global reality

Edited by John Dixon
and David Macarov

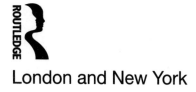

London and New York

First published 1998
by Routledge
11 New Fetter Lane, London EC4P 4EE

Simultaneously published in the USA and Canada
by Routledge
29 West 35th Street, New York, NY 10001

Typeset in Garamond by Routledge
Printed and bound in Great Britain by MPG Books Ltd, Bodmin

British Library Cataloguing in Publication Data
A catalogue record for this book is available from the British Library

Library of Congress Cataloguing in Publication Data
Poverty : a persistent global reality / edited by John Dixon and David
Macarov.
p. cm.
Includes bibliographical references and index.
1. Poverty–Case studies. 2. Poverty–Developing countries–Case
studies.
I. Dixon, John. II. Macarov, David.
HC79.P6P6816   1998
362.5–dc21   97–35431
                                                                  CIP

ISBN 0–415–14681–X (hbk)
ISBN 0–415–14682–8 (pbk)

Contents

Illustrations

Contributors

Tim Callan is a Senior Research Officer at the Economic and Social Research Institute, Dublin, Ireland.

David Cox is the Professor of Social Work at the Graduate School of Social Work, La Trobe University, Melbourne, Victoria, Australia.

Henk-Jan Dirven is in the Department of Socio-Economic Statistics of Statistics Netherlands, Amsterdam, Netherlands.

John Dixon is in the Department of Social Policy and Social Work, University of Plymouth, Plymouth, United Kingdom.

Didier Fouarge is in the Research Unit on Work and Social Security in the Work and Organisation Research Centre (WORC) at Tilburg University, Le Tilburg, Netherlands.

Karen E. Gerdes is an Assistant Professor in the School of Social Work at the Arizona State University, Temple, Arizona, United States of America.

Edwin Kaseke is the Principal of the School of Social Work, Harare, Zimbabwe.

Michelle Livermore is a Research Associate in the Office of the Research and Economic Development at Louisiana State University, Baton Rouge, Louisiana, United States of America.

David Macarov is an Emeritus Professor in the Paul Baerwald School of Social Work, at the Hebrew University, Jerusalem, Israel.

Stewart MacPherson is Professor of Development in the Centre for Development Studies, Edith Cowan University, Perth, Western Australia, Australia.

James Midgley is the Dean of the School of Social Welfare at the University of California, Berkeley, California, United States of America.

Ruud Muffels is in the Research Unit on Work and Social Security in the Work and Organisation Research Centre (WORC) at Tilburg University, Le Tilburg, Netherlands.

Brian Nolan is a Research Professor at the Economic and Social Research Institute, Dublin, Ireland.

Kyle Lynn Pehrson is a Professor and the Director of the School of Social Work at the Brigham Young University, Provo, Utah, United States of America.

Hugh Shewell is Head of the Department of Social Services and Social Work at the University College of the Fraser Valley, Abbotsford Campus, Abbotsford, British Columbia, Canada.

Richard Silburn is a Senior Lecturer in Social Policy and the Director of the Research and Postgraduate Programmes in the School of Social Studies at the University of Nottingham, Nottingham, United Kingdom.

Carmel Tabone is a Lecturer in the Department of Sociology at the University of Malta, Msida, Malta.

Preface

Poverty is one of the most ubiquitous and long-standing problems facing governments and populations throughout the world. No matter how it is defined or measured; whether in prosperous times or during depressions; whether in agricultural, industrial, or post-industrial societies; and despite anti-poverty programmes and aid to the poor, poverty continues. While poverty definitions, of course, differ as between countries, using their own country definitions, 1.1 billion people – one-fifth of the human race – live in poverty of whom 600 million are extremely poor (United Nations 1994: 76). Up to 510 million are seriously undernourished (United Nations 1990: 5). Throughout the industrialised West, the poverty rate ranges between 10 and 15 per cent of the population (Townsend 1993). In agricultural societies it is as high as 70 per cent (Bangladesh) (Townsend 1993). And in post-socialist and neo-socialist societies it is now beginning to be admitted and identified (Mroz and Popkin 1995).

This volume comprises a conceptual chapter on the meaning and measurement of poverty and ten commissioned country chapters, each of which examines, in the light of the socio-economic and historical contexts within which poverty exists, the extent and nature of poverty, its causes, and measure that have been taken to mitigate it. Each country chapter is tightly structured to facilitate comparisons. The final chapter provides a summary and conclusion.

The material included in this volume relates to early 1997. Since then, however, world events have overtaken us. Two events in particular need to be commented on. First, the consequences of the hand over of Hong Kong by the United Kingdom to China in July 1997 have not been explored, although its possible implications are dealt with. Second, the consequences of the election of a Labour government in the United Kingdom in May 1997 have also not been explored, but the poverty agenda it needs to address is well articulated.

We would like to thank all the contributors for their enthusiastic support of this volume.

To our wives, Tina and Frieda, go our thanks for putting up with our idiosyncrasies throughout the preparation of this manuscript.

For any errors of fact and for all opinions and interpretations, the authors and editors accept responsibility.

John Dixon and David Macarov
August 1997

REFERENCES

Mroz, T.A. and Popkin, B.M. (1995) 'Poverty and Economic Transition in the Russian Federation', *Economic Development and Cultural Change* 44 (1): 1–32.

Townsend, P. (1993) *The International Analysis of Poverty*, Hemel Hempstead: Harvester Wheatsheaf.

United Nations (1990) *Global Outlook 2000*, New York: United Nations.

—— (1994) *World Social Situation in the 1990s*, New York: United Nations.

Chapter 1

The meaning and measurement of poverty

Stewart MacPherson and Richard Silburn

Poverty is a persistent problem which has presented political and moral challenges to all societies at all times. The word itself, poverty, is a familiar one which everyone understands, or thinks they understand. But the specific meaning we attach to the word depends upon the underlying *concept* of poverty we have in mind. It is possible to conceptualise poverty in many different ways, each one leading towards a different understanding of the meaning and significance of the term, towards a different precise definition, which in turn will lead to parallel differences in the methods and measures used to estimate the numbers in poverty and gauge the depth of their impoverishment.

THE CONCEPTS OF POVERTY

At its simplest poverty refers to a basic lack of the means of survival; the poor are those who, even in normal circumstances, are unable to feed and clothe themselves properly and risk death as a consequence. This description would probably attract universal recognition and assent. Moreover such a situation would probably be seen as one which should if possible be rectified, although precisely how this should be done may be a matter of dispute. It is the case that there are some parts of the world where extreme poverty of this kind is prevalent and affects large numbers of people; in these cases it may be difficult in practice to argue convincingly for a less extreme concept and definition of poverty. A review of empirical studies suggests that the concept of poverty as absolute deprivation continues to be of primary relevance in countries where per capita income is low and the incidence of poverty is high.

This definition has become increasingly unacceptable in those parts of the world where higher general levels of living have been achieved. In countries experiencing rapid growth and apparent reductions in the incidence of absolute deprivation, poverty is increasingly defined in relative terms. As the threat of starvation recedes, questions concerning the appropriate distribution of income and opportunity assume greater importance. In this situation the definition of poverty moves away from a minimal, physical survival notion in the direction of a relative, varying definition which puts increasing emphasis on social survival and starts to attach value to the *quality of life* that even the poorest in a community should be able to enjoy. A different vocabulary is developed to introduce notions of social participation, of inclusion and exclusion, of citizenship, of empowerment. The idea of *relative poverty* is a powerful one, but it is also controversial, and hence the poverty debate is everywhere a hotly contested one, involving serious issues of social, political and ethical significance. In those societies where poverty is perceived to be a problem which requires remedial action of some kind, these arguments are further complicated. Is remedial action the responsibility of charitable individuals, and if so who, what and how? Is it a broader family or communal responsibility? Should the state or the government be involved and if so why and how? All of these are matters upon which people will feel entitled to have a view and therefore to disagree with one another.

Thus the first element in the analysis of poverty is to address the question of the *material level* which distinguishes the poor (those in poverty) from others. Sometimes the discussion stops altogether at this point. The problem of poverty (being poor) is presented as no more than a question of material resources, usually expressed in terms of cash. This is undoubtedly a necessary component, especially in those societies where most transactions are facilitated by transfers of cash for desired goods or services. But money for what? Any attempt to establish a poverty line expressed as a minimum cash requirement must be based upon some explicit or implicit assumptions about what that money is needed for; some sense of what needs must be addressed if the individual is not to suffer unacceptable deprivation, what goods or services it is reasonable for everyone, even the poorest, to enjoy. That this discussion is also contested reminds us that the fundamental issue is not the money itself – which has no intrinsic worth – but the effect that the lack of money has on the lives and lifestyles of the poor. A cash-deficiency definition of poverty serves as no more than a crude indicator, and to focus upon it exclusively may be to overlook other dimensions of poverty which cannot be simply reduced to monetary values. The widespread emphasis upon cash-poverty is misplaced and myopic. The concept of poverty needs to be a much fuller and more inclusive one, concerned with much more than what money can buy. It has a *moral* dimension, which, if ignored, gravely impoverishes, even distorts, any poverty debate. Fundamentally, what is offensive about poverty, and why it matters so much, is that poor people are unable to maintain a degree of control over their own lives by the exercise of *choice*. For most people daily life is a constant series of decisions and choices, from the most trivial to the most important. These choices help to fashion the quality of a person's life and that of the family to which they belong. Most choices, however, have resource implications. They involve decisions about how to use the scarce resources at one's disposal. For poor people, with few resources, the area of effective choice is constricted, and one measure of the depth of poverty is the narrowness of remaining choice.

We believe that this concept of poverty is universally defensible, although it must be interpreted sensitively. A global understanding of poverty must acknowledge that there are major cultural differences, patterns of custom and convention, of social expectation, which help to determine in any particular case the parameters within which choice is exercised, and the priorities which individuals will respond to. But it is also the case that as the extent of marketisation will vary between societies at different stages of social and economic development, so a narrow concern with cash-poverty alone without further reference to actual social and cultural situations, in all their complexity, is to engage in a discussion without real meaning.

THE DEFINITIONS OF POVERTY

Definitions of poverty will reflect the underlying concept that has been adopted, and just as poverty can be conceptualised along a continuum from the most absolute to the most relative, so there is a range of definitions (Piachaud 1987).

Subsistence poverty

The most basic definition will focus on the *capacity to survive*. In its narrowest sense this may mean nothing more than having the resources to purchase or grow sufficient food for oneself and one's dependants. The only needs that are acknowledged are biological ones, food, water, and in hostile climates, clothing and shelter. No allowances are made for broader social needs, and no recognition is given to social or cultural expectations. Using such a definition guarantees that any measure of the numbers in poverty will yield the smallest possible figure. Recommendations for policy interventions would thus be limited in scope and character, and the impact evaluation standards would be modest.

Definitions based on an *absolute* concept of poverty allow its measured prevalence to change over time. They require an absolute poverty line based on *survival* criteria, such as a specified minimum daily caloric intake (Lipton 1983) the proportion of income spent on food (Rao 1982) or the income level required to purchase some minimum basket of consumption goods.

The once common use of caloric intakes alone to determine poverty lines is in decline. It has been argued (for example, by Rodgers 1984) that the daily caloric intake is an unreliable measure of poverty. Except in unusual circumstances such as natural disasters and famines, poor people rarely die of starvation. This is partly because daily energy requirements vary with the kind and amount of activity being undertaken. Primarily, however, it is because low calorie intake has effects which are neither immediate nor necessarily measurable, for example increased susceptibility to disease. An appropriate minimum level of daily energy requirement is therefore difficult to establish.

Although isolated examples of survival definitions can still be found, it is much more commonly the case that poverty is defined by reference to some notion of *subsistence*. This certainly goes beyond mere survival, but it still a very meagre measure. It is usually based upon a basic standard of physical efficiency. Thus it might be argued that a person needs enough food not only to survive but to maintain their health at least to a level where his or her capacity to work is unimpaired. The emphasis is on purely physical needs and there is a reluctance to make any substantial acknowledgement of wider social or customary expectations and obligations.

Many attempts have been made to calculate the costs of meeting subsistence needs. One of the best-known, though often misunderstood, examples from the United Kingdom (UK) can be found in the work of Seebohm Rowntree. Rowntree endeavoured to establish a precise poverty line by drawing up a list of essential foodstuffs, and other indispensable household items, which he costed to establish an irreducible budget below which it would be difficult to maintain health and physical efficiency. In Rowntree's view this measure represented 'a standard of bare subsistence rather than living' (Rowntree 1901, 1941).

But experience has shown that even this minimalist approach to the definition of absolute poverty is, in fact, fraught with both theoretical and practical difficulties. For example, even trying to determine something as fundamental as the nutritional requirements of people of different ages or physical types is a contested matter about which dieticians and other competent experts disagree. Not only may nutritional requirements vary from one person to another, and from time to time, between people of different ages or with different work-patterns, but also, in practice, allowance may need to be made for variations in the availability of foodstuffs, in the knowledge and skills needed for the most efficient preparation of food, in food-purchasing habits where the decisions about what to buy, and in what quantity may be influenced not only by availability and price but also by capacity to store food safely and to prepare it appropriately. Beyond these important qualifications we then encounter widespread food-beliefs, dietary customs and conventions, as well as questions of taste and food-preference. All of these considerations must influence normal behaviour in ways that make the subsistence calculus much more problematic than is at first apparent.

Indeed it is clear the Rowntree himself was well aware of many of these difficulties. In his later studies he budgeted for a range of goods and services which are certainly not essential for survival or physical efficiency, but are virtually universal items of household expenditure; such as newspapers, postage stamps and trade union subscriptions (Rowntree 1941). Although this is still a very restricted budget, it is starting to recognise that there are legitimate costs which enable a person not only to survive, but to live as a member of a community within which he or she is able to take part in and contribute to normal social activities. This vividly points up the difficulties of trying to establish a living standard which excludes all but the needs of brute physical survival. In this regard we have already moved a small step towards recognising the constantly shifting and relative nature of poverty, which drives us towards definitions that start more fully to reflect this perspective.

Basic needs poverty

The *basic needs* definition of poverty is an influential variant of the subsistence model, moving somewhat towards a more relative approach. Basic needs are defined by the International Labour Organisation (1976: 7)

> [a]s the minimum standard of living which a society should set for the poorest groups of its people. The satisfaction of basic needs means
> Meeting the minimum requirements of a family for personal consumption: food, shelter, clothing; it implies access to essential services, such as safe drinking-water, sanitation, transport, health and education ... it should further imply the satisfaction of needs of a more qualitative nature: a healthy, humane and satisfying environment, and popular participation in the making of decisions.

Indeed, the achievement in each country of a certain specific minimum standard of living became a major policy recommendation of the International Labour Organisation in 1976.

The major importance of basic needs concept is that it is not confined to the physical needs for individual survival, but recognises the importance of a range of community services and facilities, often of an infrastructural kind, and beyond these some non-material qualitative assets. It recognises that the basic needs objectives will vary from one country to another in the light of specific circumstances,

> levels of development, climatic conditions, social and cultural values. Basic needs are therefore in large part a relative concept; but there are also certain minimum levels of personal consumption and access to social services which should be universally regarded as essential to a decent life.
> (International Labour Organisation 1976: 7)

To operationalise basic needs raises many of the same difficulties that we have observed with reference to subsistence measures. Important, difficult and inescapable value-judgements have to be made, in the context of each country's social and economic circumstances, to establish the criteria and components of basic needs, and to measure progress towards their attainment.

By now it is clear that the attempt to construct an absolute and presumably universal definition of poverty is fundamentally flawed, both in theory and practice. Poverty analysts are driven remorselessly to accept that poverty has to be understood as a socially constructed concept with powerful qualitative and normative components. As such it is inherently a *relative* concept.

Relative poverty

All relative definitions of poverty are based upon comparison, often with some notion of prevailing living standards in the community being researched. Thus one might examine prevailing patterns of expenditure and consumption and define as poor those whose '[i]ncomes or resources are not sufficient to provide them with those goods and services that will enable them to live a life that is tolerable according to working-class life-styles' (George and Howards 1991: 6).

A broadly similar approach to relative poverty from the Council of Ministers of the European Community in 1984 defined the poor as '[p]ersons, families and groups of persons whose resources (material, cultural and social) are so limited as to exclude them from the minimum acceptable way of life in the Member State in which they live' (Council of the European Communities 1984, Council Decision on Specific Community Action to Combat Poverty 85/8/EEC). Although this definition is imprecise the thrust is clear enough, and is based upon a comparison with some measure of prevailing living standards.

Peter Townsend's views on 'relative deprivation' go rather further than this, and stress the importance of 'social participation'. In *Poverty in the United Kingdom* (1979) he conceptualised relative poverty as one where material consumption and social participation in a wide range of customary social activities is inhibited by lack of resources. More recently he has suggested:

Poverty may be best understood as applying . . . to those whose resources do not allow them to fulfil the elaborate social demands and customs which have been placed upon citizens of that society . . . . If people lack or are denied resources to obtain access to diets, amenities, standards, services, and activities which are common or customary in society, or to meet the obligations expected of them or imposed upon them in their social roles and relationships and so fulfil membership of society, they may be said to be in poverty.

(Townsend 1993: 36)

Adopting a relative definition of poverty certainly complicates the research and policy process, in theoretical and practical ways. Theoretically, there is likely to be disagreement about the appropriate levels for comparison, and at the practical level it assumes a considerable volume of accurate and regularly up-dated information about income and consumption patterns. In many places this information is simply not available or is unreliable, and policy-makers must look elsewhere. But as a critical concept relative poverty points us in the right direction and gives us a yardstick by which progress can be evaluated.

THE MEASUREMENT OF POVERTY

If serious research is to be undertaken into the extent and nature of poverty, or if policies are to be developed that try to reduce the extent of poverty, then reliable and relevant *measures* need to be developed that will enable us to determine how many poor there are in any given population and what are the social characteristics of the poor (for example, their gender, ages, family circumstances and work-experience).

There is a wide range of possible measures that have been developed and deployed in different countries. As we would expect the kind of measure chosen reflects the underlying concept and definition of poverty that has been adopted. If the chosen measure has been adopted by responsible public authorities to help make informed policy decisions then the measure will also reflect the dominant prevailing ideology of social policy. It will also be influenced by the availability of appropriate and reliable social data which can be used as the basis for the calculation.

Most research and policy-making takes place within specific countries, and consequently many of the measures to be described are national ones. Recently, however, there has been growing interest in the possibility of developing cross-national and international measures so that legitimate comparisons can be made between one country or group of countries and another.

The Orshansky scale and basic needs

The first set of measures are related to a concept of poverty which is close to the subsistence model. An individual or family are poor if they lack the resources to sustain an acceptable, but low, level of social living: the minimum standard of living which a society should set for the poorest groups of its people. How has this definition been developed into a measure?

The United States (US) is one of the few countries which has developed an official poverty line, which is widely understood and used:

> Poverty statistics published by the Bureau of the Census are used in a variety of ways. The media use such numbers to compare trends in poverty over time and differences in poverty among such groups as the elderly and children. Government agencies . . . use the poverty threshold . . . in targeting services and resources to disadvantaged persons . . . academic researchers use the concept as a measure of individual and family well-being.
> (Institute for Research on Poverty 1995: 2)

The poverty line was developed in the early 1960s by Molly Orshansky, an economist working for the Social Security Administration, and was adopted as an official threshold by the US federal government (Orshansky 1969). The Orshansky approach is a widely-used compromise between nutritional and income-based methods for establishing poverty lines. It is calculated by first finding the minimum expenditure required to satisfy nutritional requirements, then 'grossing up' this figure by an appropriate proportion to allow for non-food expenditure requirements. In this way the Orshansky approach incorporates the view that poverty has a social as well as a biological dimension. The thresholds set in 1963 have been updated annually since then to take account of price inflation. This means that the 1963 purchasing power has been maintained in real terms, but there has been no further adjustments to reflect other major changes in living standards, and in consumption and expenditure patterns.

The merit of such a poverty-threshold is that it is clear, and relatively easily calculated and amended. The disadvantage is that it is a single and crude measure which will take no account of the many pressures that face poorer people. An official panel set up in 1992 to review the measure, recommended a number of changes which will make the measure much more sensitive, but it will still be based upon a measurable minimum level of acceptable living. The principal recommendation was that

> the official poverty thresholds should comprise a budget for the three basic categories of food, clothing and shelter, plus a little more. Certain non-discretionary expenditures such as taxes, child-care and other costs associated with working and medical costs should be treated as deductions from income. Thresholds would be updated with reference not simply to price changes, but to changes in the pattern of consumption of food, clothing and shelter; resources to include gross money-income plus the value of near-money benefits in kind (such as food stamps). [The new measure] more effectively targets benefits to needy families . . . it reflects geographic differences in the cost of housing, and its definition of family resources . . . is consistent with the basic needs concept underlying the thresholds.
>
> (Institute for Research on Poverty 1995: 8)

Budget standards

The budget standards technique is a method of assessing poverty which has recently enjoyed a revival of interest after a long period of neglect. Essentially a poverty line would be determined by reference to the calculated cost of an agreed basket of goods. In essence this was the method adopted by Rowntree at the beginning of the century to calculate an absolute poverty line as a *standard of bare subsistence rather than living*. But the technique can be used in a much less restrictive manner. For example, countries where there is a regular family expenditure survey could derive the basket of goods by reference to the evidence of how families of different composition and income levels actually spend their income, and could vary the content of the basket of goods in the light of evidence of changing spending patterns.

Recent work carried out at the University of York has developed a range of so-called modest-but-adequate budgets for families of different sizes and compositions (Bradshaw and Ernst 1990; Bradshaw *et al.* 1987). A 'less-eligible' version of this budget, a 'low-cost' budget, has also been elaborated, and this has been used in the UK as one way of evaluating the adequacy or otherwise of benefit-levels. A similar approach was adopted in a research project recently completed in Hong Kong. This study compiled a set of budgets based upon the evidence about actual expenditure patterns in Hong Kong, reinforced by survey evidence about the circumstances of benefit-claimants. More recent work in Hong Kong has extended the basis for assessing actual expenditure through a household survey (see Chapter 4, Hong Kong).

Developing and costing what is considered to be an acceptable basket of goods is in practice very difficult, and involves the exercise of considerable judgement, especially when there is a definite move beyond agreed items to consider other kinds of expenditure, such as transport costs for social reasons, leisure and cultural activities, or fulfilling socially required family obligations. There is a powerful case for extending the range of items included to encompass housing, domestic commodities and ownership of other assets (see Chapter 6, Malta). Sherraden (1991: 293) argues that both concepts of poverty, and the policies designed to respond to poverty, should focus more strongly on assets rather than income:

> Asset accumulation and investment, rather than income and consumption, are the keys to leaving poverty. Therefore welfare policy should promote asset accumulation – stake holding – by the poor. An asset-based welfare policy would seek to combine welfare assistance with economic development.

Public opinion and social consensus measures

The considerable problems which arise from reliance on expert judgement in the definition and implementation of poverty measures has led to a number of efforts to find a broader basis for support for the components of a poverty line. These approaches seek to define and measure the extent of poverty by reference to the views of the general public rather than the judgement of a group of experts. As Piachaud (1987: 149), this is an effort 'to cast aside self-appointed, self-opinionated experts' and 'let the people decide'. There are a number of variants on the consensus approach. Some obtain views about hypothetical families (Rainwater 1974), while others focus on respondents' views about their own situation or how much income they need (Goedhart *et al.* 1977; see also Malta (Chapter 6) and the Netherlands (Chapter 7)).

Another consensus approach consists of asking which components of living standards are 'necessary' (Mack and Lansley 1985). They sought to 'identify a minimum acceptable way of life not by reference to the views of "experts", nor by reference to observed patterns of expenditure or observed living standards, but by reference to the view of society as a whole' (p. 43).

Their study defined deprivation in terms of 'an enforced lack of socially perceived necessities' (p. 41). Depravations were only termed 'poverty' when they affect a person's way of life. This approach was based upon a general survey of households in which respondents were asked about which items they regarded as necessities, which all adults should be able to afford and which they should not have to do without. Respondents were also asked about items which might be desirable but not necessary. The Mack and Lansley study has been summarised by Saunders and Matheson (1992: 20):

> The survey instrument included a list of thirty-five goods, services and activities and respondents were asked which of these they would classify as 'necessities'. Items chosen were intended as indicators of 'not only the basic essentials for survival (such as food) but also access or otherwise, to participating in society and being able to play a social role . . . .' From these items, Mack and Lansley found 22 which were rated as necessities by a majority of their sample and whose absence was negatively correlated with income. They then proceeded to classify as poor anyone who could not afford three or more of them. This was translated into an income level by means of fitting regression equations to the data for low and high income families to see if there was any given point at which the relationship between income and deprivation significantly diverged.

But the method has been criticised because people's responses are firmly based on their own subjective experience, which may be far removed from the poverty level. It is also problematic who selects the list of items deemed to be indicative of the way of life of a particular society (Ashton 1984; Piachaud 1987; Viet-Wilson 1987).

In an attempt to overcome some of these problems other

researchers have sought to ask respondents directly about the adequacy or inadequacy of given income levels. The subjective poverty line (SPL) and the Leyden poverty line (LPL) are, according to Kapteyn *et al.* (1988: 222) 'both subjective in that they are based on responses to survey questions which try to elicit a respondent's evaluation of the income levels or his/her judgement about minimum needs'.

The SPL is based on responses to questions on what income levels the respondents consider to be the minimum they themselves need to make ends meet (Goedhart *et al.* 1977; Flick and van Praag 1991; van den Bosch *et al.* 1993; Saunders, Hallerod and Matheson 1992). The LPL is based on the concept of the welfare function of income. Poverty is seen as, according to Goedhart *et al.* (1977: 504):

> a situation in which the consumption set of individuals is severely constricted, while affluence is defined as a situation in which there is little constriction of the consumption set . . . [poverty is] a situation where command over resources falls below a certain level, the poverty line.

The method based on this approach uses income evaluation questions, which essentially ask how much income respondents judge their households need to meet various levels of satisfaction. But people may not be able to judge the income needed for a particular standard of living, and may vary in their interpretation of key notions such as 'making ends meet'. There can be dramatically different answers in responses to only slight changes in the wording of questions (Walker 1987; Hagenaars and de Vos 1988; van den Bosch *et al.* 1993).

Another approach in the consensus tradition is that which *uses hypothetical family techniques*. An example of this is the Gallop Poll question that asks 'what is the smallest amount of money a family of four needs to get along in your community?' (Danziger *et al.* 1984: 501). Rainwater (1974) extended this approach to encompass different levels of living and household composition. Dubnoff (1986) developed a technique that is a variant of this, in which respondents are asked to rate, according to scale, the level of living of hypothetical families with varying incomes and other characteristics. This approach does obtain respondents' views on a range of household. Although public opinion and social consensus approaches can contribute a great deal, they face a serious conceptual and practical problem, which, according to Saunders and Matheson (1992: 25) lies in 'expecting respondents to estimate an appropriate income for someone whose circumstances and/or preferences may be completely unlike their own. They have to judge what given income level would mean for someone else.'

Benefit dependency measures

In many countries, and especially those which have well-developed social security systems, the number of people who are receiving benefits, particularly those who are long-term recipients, is often used as another measure of poverty. At one level this is a curious idea. It could be argued that the purpose of social security is precisely to lift people out of poverty, and so an estimate of those in receipt of benefits should indicate not those in poverty, but on the contrary, the number whose poverty has been mitigated. It could also be argued, of course, that benefit rates may be set at a very low rate, well below average earnings, and thus do not provide an acceptable poverty threshold measure. The budget standard method has recently been used in England (Family Budget Unit 1992) to demonstrate that for many recipient groups the current levels of social assistance do not permit even a *modest-but-adequate* lifestyle. From this perspective the level of benefit payment represents a threshold below which it is deemed unsuitable for anyone to be expected to live, and thus significant changes in the numbers and composition of long-term claimants is a clear indication of poverty trends.

Household expenditure measures

Measures of relative poverty using household expenditure have become increasingly widespread in recent years. This measure is only possible where there is reliable and regularly up-dated information in sufficient detail of patterns of household expenditure. This often takes the form of an annual official survey of household expenditure patterns. Thus in the UK, since 1988, a measure called the *Households Below Average Income* (HBAI) draws upon the Family Expenditure Survey and has become a major source of official data about people on low incomes (UK, DSS 1995). In this case the annual Family Expenditure Survey permits the participating households to be ranked, and then a cut-off point is chosen to mark a poverty-threshold. This is sometimes set as low as 40 per cent of the mean average household income, but more usually 50 per cent is the preferred cut-off. Strictly speaking this is not so much a poverty measure as a measure of relative inequality. However, the use of a HBAI figure produces a poverty estimate that is very similar to that obtained when using benefit-levels as the base-line. Above all, as many countries now conduct regular expenditure surveys, this method has at least the potential of enabling the poverty situation to be compared between countries as well as within them. This is an important point as international and cross-national comparisons become more widely sought after. A sophisticated recent example from Europe compared patterns of poverty in the twelve countries of the European Union using standardised data from national Household Budget Surveys. The definition of poverty used was a relative one, and data was presented using three cut-off points at 40 per cent, 50 per cent and 60 per cent of average expenditure, believing that expenditure information was more accurately reported than income data.

Household expenditure measures do, of course, have their limita-tions. Crucially, they depend upon the quality of the data from which they are derived. Household surveys certainly exclude those people who are not members of households, such as the homeless or those in institutions. Furthermore, reliable income data is difficult to collect, and household expenditure figures do not reflect access to non-cash resources which, in some circumstances, may make a considerable contribution to living standards, nor do they capture the effect on family well-being of tax-financed, state-provided goods and services (such as health care or education).

Further issues of definition concern the units over which poverty is measured. In practice, most empirical studies take the household as their basic unit of analysis, for the practical reason that this is usually the lowest level to which income and expenditure can be disaggregated in developing country data. This approach implicitly assumes that expenditure is distributed within the household in such a way as to provide equal satisfaction of needs, and, usually, that the composition of households of the same size is invariant between poor and non-poor. An analysis by Bhalla and Vashistha (1988) explores the potential variation in poverty estimates that can arise due to the adoption of different definitions of an 'average household'.

Because poor families are larger, the number of households in poverty will invariably be substantially lower than the number of individuals unless suitable weights are employed in constructing the measure. For example, Anand (1983: 127) reported for Malaysia in the early 1970s that 'while the percentage of persons in poverty is 40.2 per cent, the percentage of households in poverty is 36.5 per cent. This is because the poor have larger average household size than the non-poor.'

Another discussion of the problem in an empirical context can be found in Meesook (1976). It is generally rare for sufficient information to be available to investigate and correct for variation in household composition in a rigorous manner.

CONCLUSION

Being poor is a complex and wide-ranging state. It is affected by many factors including income, health, education, access to goods, location, gender, race and family circumstances. We know that it is very difficult to measure poverty in such a way as to express this complex multidimensional quality. Commonly, income and/or expenditure are used to measure poverty, but in all countries it is important to consider many other indicators of the quality of life. The most basic are life expectancy, infant mortality and school enrolment rates. All these are important in themselves, but also act powerfully as expressions of the state of social conditions. Our discussion is restricted largely to indicators of income and expenditure. To make any meaningful statements about poverty conditions or trends internationally we must have data that is comparable.

There is considerable data now available for high income countries that allows sophisticated comparison between countries, between groups within countries and regions, and over time. For the low and middle income countries, the situation is much less good. But in recent years the amount and the quality of data have improved a great deal. In 1993 there were only eleven countries with household survey based data on income and/or consumption expenditures. In 1996 there were forty-four (World Bank 1996: 2). Unfortunately, the poorer a country is, the less likely it is to have data collection capability, and the lower the quality of any data that is collected, and the less relevant measures of cash are going to be as indicators of levels of living. Because of the paucity of data many studies of poverty have used synthetic estimates of country poverty rates based upon whatever survey observations are available together with assumptions drawn widely from relevant and comparable circumstances elsewhere (World Bank 1995). These are very crude. Add to this that even when there is survey data, the measures used vary greatly, and clearly international comparison is very difficult indeed. Several international agencies have sought to produce a consistent poverty line that allows comparisons to be made. The latest World Bank research on poverty for example uses US$1 per day (converted to local currency to reflect local prices) as a *minimum poverty line* (World Bank 1996). The data produced using this measure is based on survey data from the countries concerned. Thus the US$1 per day line is quite arbitrary. It has been adopted to enable comparison, to allow measurement at different places and different times, thus allowing comparisons to be made, and trends assessed.

Poverty is the most serious social problem facing the international community. As we have seen, although the specific content of poverty definitions will vary between countries, the essential nature of poverty as a condition is universal. Poverty is about exclusion. It is a wide-ranging and complex phenomenon, profoundly affecting individuals and households. The emphasis on exclusion directs us to the heart of poverty: that the lack of resources prevents participation in the normal life of the community. The particular form of those resources will be different in different communities, as will the notions of what constitutes a normal lifestyle. The fundamental concept is simple, but operationalising it is complex, and profoundly political.

Our concept of poverty determines our definition, and our definition determines our measures. What we choose to measure, and how, gives us the problem we choose to confront, and thus shapes our policy. We have seen that the seemingly academic questions of poverty – definition and measurement – have profound consequences for policy and practice, and thus for those now condemned to poverty and its consequences. Unless and until the poverty problem is adequately conceptualised, defined and measured, countless millions will continue to suffer.

REFERENCES

Anand, S. (1983) *Poverty and Inequality in Malaysia: Measurement and Decomposition*, New York: Oxford University Press for the World Bank.

Ashton, P. (1984) 'Poverty and its Beholders', *New Society* 70/10139: 95–8
Bhalla, S.S. and Vashistha, P.S. (1988) 'Income Distribution in India: A Re-examination', in Srinivasan, J. and Bardhan, H. (eds) *Rural Poverty in South Asia*, New York: Columbia University Press.
Bosch, K. van den, Callen, T., Estivill, J., Hausman, P., Jeanddidier, B., Muffels, R. and Yantopoulos, J. (1993) 'A Comparison of Poverty in Seven European Countries and Regions Using Subjective and Relative Measures', *Journal of Population Economics* 6 (1): 235–59.
Bradshaw, J. and Ernst, J. (1990) *Establishing a Modest-but-adequate Budget for a British Family*, York: Joseph Rowntree.
Bradshaw J., Mitchell, D. and Morgan, J. (1987) 'Evaluating Adequacy: The Potential of Budget Standards', *Journal of Social Policy* 16 (2): 189–215.
Danziger, S., van der Gaag, J., Taussig, M.K. and Smolensky, E. (1984) 'The Direct Measurement of Welfare Levels: How Much is Cost to make Ends Meet?', *Review of Economics and Statistics* 66 (3): 500–5.
Dubnoff, S. (1986) 'How Much is Enough', *Public Opinion Quarterly* 49 (2): 285–99.
Family Budget Unit (1992) *Household Budgets and Living Standards* (Social Policy Research Findings No. 32), York: Joseph Rowntree Foundation.
Flick, R.J. and van Praag, B.M.S. (1991) 'Subjective Poverty Line Definitions', *De Economist* 139 (3): 311–30.
George, V. and Howards, I. (1991) *Poverty Amidst Affluence*, Aldershot: Edward Elgar.
Goedhart, T., Halberstadt, V., Kapteyn, A. and van Preaag, B.M.S. (1977) 'The Poverty Line: Concepts and Measurements', *Journal of Human Resources* 12 (4): 503–20.
Hagenaars, A. and Vos, K. de (1988) 'The Definition and Measurement of Poverty', *The Journal of Human Resources* 22 (2): 211–21.
Institute for Research on Poverty (1995) *Bulletin* 17 (1), Madison: University of Wisconsin.
International Labour Organisation (ILO) (1976) *Meeting Basic Needs: Strategies for Eradicating Mass Poverty and Unemployment*, Geneva: ILO.
Kapteyn, A., Kooreman, P. and Willemse, R. (1988) 'Some Methodological Issues in the Implementation of Subjective Poverty Definitions', *Journal of Human Resources* 22 (2): 222–42
Lipton, M. (1983) *Poverty, Undernutrition and Hunger* (Staff Working Papers No. 597), Washington, DC: World Bank.
Mack, J. and Lansley, S. (1985), *Poor Britain*, London: George, Allen and Unwin.
Meesook, O.A. (1976) *Income Distribution in Thailand* (Discussion Paper No. 76–12), Diliman, Quezon City: Council for Asian Manpower Studies.
Orshansky, M (1969) 'How Poverty is Measured', *Monthly Labour Review* 92 (2): 37–41.
Piachaud, D. (1987) 'Problems in the Definition and Measurement of Poverty', *Journal of Social Policy* 16 (2): 147–64.
Rainwater, L. (1974) *What Money Buys: Inequality and the Social Meaning of Income*, New York: Basic Books.

Rao, V. (1982) *Food, Nutrition and Poverty in India*, Hemel Hempstead: Harvester Wheatsheaf.

Rodgers, G. (1984) *Poverty and Population: Approaches and Evidence*, Geneva: ILO.

Rowntree, S. (1901) *Poverty: a Study of Town Life*, London: Macmillan.

—— (1941) *Poverty and Progress*, London: Longmans, Green.

Saunders, P. and Bradbury, B. (1991) 'Some Australian Evidence on the Consensual Approach to Poverty Measurement', *Economic Analysis and Policy* 21 (1): 47–78.

Saunders, P. and Matheson, G. (1992) *Perceptions of Poverty, Income Adequacy and Living Standards in Australia* (Reports and Proceedings No. 99), Sydney: Social Policy Research Centre, University of New South Wales.

Saunders, P., Hallerod, B. and Matheson, G. (1992) 'Making Ends Meet in Australia and Sweden: A Comparative Analysis Using the Subjective Poverty Line Methodology', *Acta Sociologica* 37 (1): 3–22.

Sherraden, M.W. (1991) *Assets and the Poor*, New York: Sharpe.

Townsend, P. (1979) *Poverty in the United Kingdom*, Harmondsworth: Penguin.

—— (1993) *The International Analysis of Poverty*, Hemel Hempstead: Harvester Wheatsheaf.

United Kingdom, Department of Social Security (UK, DSS) (1995) *Households Below Average Income: A Statistical Analysis*, London: HMSO.

Viet-Wilson, J.H. (1987) 'Consensual Approaches to Poverty Lines and Social Security', *Journal of Social Policy* 16 (2): 183–211.

Walker, R. (1987) 'Consensual Approaches to the Definition of Poverty: Towards an Alternative Methodology', *Journal of Social Policy* 16 (2): 212–26.

World Bank (1995) *Social Indicators Report 1995*, Baltimore: Johns Hopkins University Press.

—— (1996) *Poverty Reduction and the World Bank: Progress and Challenges in the 1990s*, Washington, DC: The World Bank.

Chapter 2

Australia

David Cox

Australia is a large sparsely-populated island continent, with an area of 7,687 square kilometres, of which only 8 per cent is arable land, and has a population of just over eighteen million people. One-third of the country is not suited to economic development.

The early history of Australia goes back at least 18,000 years when the Aboriginal peoples are believed to have arrived across a land bridge from Asia. Modern history began in 1770 with the arrival of Captain Cook who claimed the country for England. In 1787 England began to send out prisoners (convicts) who, together with the military who guarded them, officials and earlier settlers, founded a network of colonies. In 1901 these colonies were federated into the Commonwealth of Australia, comprised of five states and two territories.

Australia's eighteen million people are concentrated in three coastal regions – the east, south-east and south-west seaboards, none of which extend more than 300 kilometres inland. Australia is one of the most urbanised countries in the world. By 1976, some 86 per cent of the population were living in urban centres, which has changed but little since. It is also a very concentrated form of urbanisation, with 54 per cent of the population living in five urban centres.

The total population is growing at the very slow rate of 1.1 per cent (1990–4 average), contributed to by migration. In total, five million immigrants arrived in Australia between 1945 and 1991, of whom the great majority have remained. This has given the country one of the world's highest proportions of overseas-born – about 21 per cent. In addition, a further 20 per cent are the children of overseas-born parents.

As with many other Western countries, Australia has an ageing population. The fertility rate has fallen in recent decades to around 1.8, and the proportion aged 65 and over reached 11.4 per cent in 1991. It is predicted to reach 20 per cent by the year 2031. Accordingly, the dependency ratio has declined quite markedly since 1971, but should bottom out early in the next century.

Economically Australia is a comparatively wealthy industrialised country. Its Gross Domestic Product per capita is A$25,975 (1995) and most Australians enjoy a high standard of living. The country is ranked eleventh on the United Nations Development Program's Human Development Index. It has a life expectancy of 77 and a high performance overall on all major social indicators. This performance, however, does conceal a very poor situation among the Aboriginal population (numbering some 284,000 in 1991), a growing gap between rich and poor and some serious social problems.

The country is well endowed with minerals, and its economic growth has depended in part on the export of iron ore, coal, uranium, bauxite and other minerals. The other major area of exports has been agricultural products, and particularly wool and wheat. Its abundant natural gas reserves, hydroelectric potential and coal resources have represented a further boost to economic growth. Manufacturing saw major development in the post-war decades, aided by immigration, but more recently service industries have grown greatly in significance.

In the period 1985–94 Australia experienced an average growth rate of 1.2 per cent, and currently has low inflation and interest rates, but this situation continues to be marred by high unemployment levels – 8.7 per cent overall in 1996, but some 20 per cent for youth. In recent years considerable effort has gone into raising education participation levels, but the percentage moving into tertiary education, around 50 per cent, is still considered to be too low.

Given its still considerable reliance on primary commodity exports Australia remains vulnerable to volatile international markets in this area. Its location, climatic conditions and population size may still have some adverse consequences in economic performance; and immigration as a source of expansion is today more controversial than it has ever been before. Given these various conditions and Australia's place in international systems, it may be unwise to assume that Australia's major strategy in tackling poverty lies in continuing economic growth. Important though that may be, the indicators are that it may do little to alter the causes, and therefore the incidence of poverty.

THE APPROPRIATE DEFINITION OF POVERTY

The only populations in Australia that can be associated with absolute poverty are the Aborigines and those who, because of homelessness, are unable to fit the requirements of income-support schemes. Among the latter population are homeless youth, derelict men, and a proportion of the deinstitutionalised population. The reasons for absolute poverty within these two populations are both different and varied.

The more generally applicable definition of poverty in Australia is relative poverty, usually defined in terms similar to that articulated by Davidson and Lees (1993: 1): 'Individuals in society may be considered to be living in poverty when they are unable to access the resources they require for participating in the normal living patterns and activities of the society of which they are part.'

Poverty in Australia is commonly considered, according to Taylor and McClelland (1994: 4): 'principally in terms of lack of economic resources, most easily measured and described in terms of lack of money (low income) and how that prevents people from obtaining a decent standard of living and from participation in society'.

It is a small step, however, to move from an inadequate level of income in a relative poverty context, to the issue of income inequality generally. There is great concern in Australia, as expressed by Saunders (1994: 191)

> that increased inequality has occurred as a result of the end of the long economic boom of the 1950s and 1960s, the fiscal crisis that this produced, and the resulting attempts by governments throughout the industrialised world to rationalise welfare programmes and deregulate the economy.

Elsewhere, Saunders (1993: 40) links the considerable increase in income inequality between 1981–2 and 1989–90 with a rise in relative poverty. For many writers this focus on inequality is crucial because it implies a focus on structural inequality as the major cause of inequality of outcome – whether of opportunity, income or access to goods and services (see, for example, Harris 1989: 7). However, in a recent very detailed study of inequality in Australia, Johnson, Manning and Hellwig (1995: 24) acknowledge that 'there is a common perception in Australia that economic inequality has increased over the last fifteen years', but conclude (p. 24):

The results suggest that while market determined inequality has increased this has been more than counter balanced by government intervention . . . . Overall . . . there appears to have been an appreciable fall in inequality over the period [1981–94] as a whole when measured by equivalised social wage income.

This logical discussion of the meaning of poverty in the Australian context results in a dilemma when it comes to measurement. Relative poverty and inequality both point to a range of indicators of poverty. For example, a major indicator of income-related poverty may be as much the security and stability of the income flow as the quantity of income received (Ternowetsky 1980); or attitudes like a sense of powerlessness might be important; or the quality of housing and the general standard of living in material terms might be the critical factor. In relation to the Aboriginal population, Choo (1990: 10) identified, from a consultation approach, that

the emphasis was placed on a non-material view of poverty, on issues pertaining to relationships, reciprocal obligations and responsibilities or the breakdown in these relationships, as well as the deeply spiritual link with the environment and each other . . . . They were saddened by the loss of social order and disintegration of their communities, the loss of identity, self-respect and a sense of control over their own destiny and future. It was clear that poverty was given a much broader definition than the usual definition in the literature.

Despite this sense of a wide range of indicators of poverty reflecting complex situations and structural contexts giving rise to poverty, when it came to the measurement of poverty almost invariably the strategy used has been a poverty line known as the 'Henderson poverty line', which is basically an income measurement applied in a relatively arbitrary fashion. In other words, such a measure bears little resemblance to actual needs and costs, and ignores the non-income dimensions of poverty. Its use also carries the danger that the implied solution to poverty is invariably to increase people's income, which ignores structural and other factors.

The Henderson poverty line was the product of a Commission of Inquiry into Poverty, chaired by Professor Ronald Henderson, which reported in 1975 (Australia, Commission of Inquiry into Poverty

1975). It used a poverty line to measure the extent of poverty and, despite the considerable controversy surrounding this poverty line, it has been used since 1975 in a variety of ways. The poverty line depends on three main definitions: a definition of a poverty threshold level of income; a definition of the income unit among which that income is assumed to be shared; and an equivalence scale to adjust it for the different costs of living of income units of different size.

The poverty line was initially set as equal to the minimum wage plus family benefits for a one-earner couple with two children. This minimum wage bore little relationship to needs or costs but to the nation's capacity (or willingness) to pay. It was, however, readily capable of being indexed to national average weekly earnings (Carter 1991: 15–19). Because of the obvious relevance of housing costs, the 1975 Henderson Poverty Inquiry went on to introduce a second poverty line, to be applied after housing costs were deducted from income.

The standard unit sharing an income was husband, wife and two children. This definition became less and less valid as the numbers of one-parent households increased dramatically.

Finally, in the absence of any reliable Australian equivalence scale, the Henderson Poverty Inquiry used the 1954 Family Budgets Standards devised in New York. This too has been strongly criticised as inappropriate but has never been replaced. Why the relative cost of living for a man and a woman, an adult and child, a boy and girl and so on which applied in New York in 1954 would resemble the (in any case diverse) Australian situation in 1975 or 1996 is a mystery.

While the Australian approach to the measurement of poverty is not consistent with many of the detailed definitions of poverty, nor an approach which is beyond criticism, it is the approach which has been used since 1966, and has at least the advantage of consistency.

THE INCIDENCE OF POVERTY

Using the poverty line described above, the 1975 Henderson Poverty Inquiry (1975: 14) found the following to be the incidence of poverty:

Our overall measure of poverty, in terms of adult income units, shows that on an annual income basis, 10.2 per cent were 'very poor' (below 100 per cent of the poverty line) and 7.7 per cent were 'rather poor' (between 100 per cent and 120 per cent of the poverty line).

It was held by the Henderson Poverty Inquiry (p. 27), and widely agreed, that the poverty line drawn was austere. We can compare these results with those obtained in a 1966 study, which revealed that the incidence of poverty was then 7.7 per cent 'very poor' for Melbourne only, while the comparable Melbourne figure in 1973 was 7.3 per cent (Henderson, Harcourt and Harper 1970). Poverty emerged as a serious social issue in Australia only in the 1970s (Graycar and Jamrozik 1993: 30). In the aftermath of the 1975 Henderson Poverty Inquiry, and because of the changes which occurred in Australia's economic conditions, the situation was closely studied. The Henderson poverty line framework was applied to the data available from the 1990 Survey of Income and Housing Costs and Amenities, which was conducted by the Australian Bureau of Statistics and the analysis was carried out by the Social Policy Research Centre at the University of New South Wales. Estimates were made of the situation both before and after housing costs. The overall poverty incidence was 16.4 per cent before housing and 15.0 per cent after housing. The respective figures in 1981–2 had been 10.2 and 9.4 per cent. There was a clear and significant increase in the overall incidence of poverty during the 1980s. As Saunders (1993: 39) comments:

The 1980s saw a combination of two factors in Australia which might have been expected to lead to reductions in both income inequality and poverty. The first was the existence for much of the decade of a government committed to equity and social justice. The second was the performance of the economy, at least between 1983 and 1989 which, while not spectacular relative to that achieved in the 1950s and 1960s, was moderately successful particularly in terms of employment growth.

The reality of a rising incidence of poverty in a context of economic growth and a sympathetic government has to be grounds for real concern. What, according to Saunders (1994: 143),

needs to be emphasised, however, [is] that the growth in average incomes over the period resulted in the real value of the Henderson poverty line increasing by some 9 per cent between

1981–82 and 1989–90 . . . . This highlights the fact that the trends in relative poverty . . . reveal a more fundamental change over the decade, the increase in income inequality.

Saunders (p. 146) goes on to suggest that this situation was widespread internationally, which 'casts serious doubt on the "trickle down" theory of redistribution which argues that the most effective way to improve the circumstances of the poor is through economic growth which raises incomes overall'.

Although the increase in overall poverty has occurred across all sections of the Australian population, it is nonetheless important not only to identify the groups which are most affected by poverty but also to understand why this is so.

GROUPS MOST AFFECTED BY POVERTY

The most important point to recognise in considering which groups are most affected by poverty is the centrality of employment. As the 1975 Henderson Poverty Inquiry states (Australia, Commission of Inquiry into Poverty 1975: 16):

the dominant factor which determines poverty is whether or not the head of the income unit is able to work. The 1973 survey showed that the great majority of the very poor were not in the workforce, and a much larger proportion of those not in the workforce were poorer than of those in the workforce.

One can then go further, as the Henderson Poverty Inquiry does, and distinguish the specific categories of people who are more likely to be found in poverty. In terms of the 'very poor' (below the poverty line), aged single males and fatherless families were the two categories which dominated, with aged single females following close behind. The percentage in poverty for each of these groups was 36.6, 36.5 and 31.0 respectively, which is nearly 10 percentage points beyond the next most vulnerable group – the sick or invalid with 21.4 per cent. The situation was also virtually unchanged in terms of ranking when one combined the 'very poor' and 'rather poor' – under and within 20 per cent of the poverty line. What did change the situation dramatically, however, was taking the cost of housing into account. After housing, the fatherless families were by far the most likely to be in poverty, with 30.0 per cent, while the unemployed and the sick and invalid followed with 18.7 and 17.9 per cent respectively.

All of the above poverty incidence data on those categories of people most likely to be in poverty refer to adult income units. If one used, instead, persons in poverty as the unit, the Henderson Poverty Inquiry found that 'there are more children in poverty after housing than there are adults because many families are worst off when this measure is used' (Australia, Commission of Inquiry into Poverty 1975: 15). By contrast, aged persons tend to be better off after housing.

Some ten years later, using 1985–6 figures, the single-parent income unit emerges as the most likely to be in poverty, with 54.5 per cent before and 43.5 per cent after housing, compared with overall figures of 17.7 and 12.4 per cent. Next most likely to be in poverty were married couples with four or more children (40.7 and 31.0 per cent before and after housing), followed by single persons over 65 years of age, with 30.6 and 5.6 per cent. These three groups dominated the poverty profile of the mid-1980s (see Harris 1989).

From these data on income units in poverty flow two unmistakable, alarming and frequently referred to conclusions. One is that the number of children in poverty had virtually tripled in the 1970s and 1980s, with some 20 per cent under an austere poverty line. The other is that 'households headed by women have continued to be four to five times as likely to be poor as those headed by men' (Harris 1989: 6). There was absolutely no doubt that in Australia 'the burden of poverty was falling disproportionately on the young' (Crossley 1990: 1) and that sole-parent families were highly vulnerable, especially when headed by women. The overall incidence of poverty among sole parent families was placed at 56 per cent in 1986 (Morris and Trethewey 1988: iv) – a disturbingly high figure. And of course the children of such families suffered accordingly: '65 per cent of Australian children in sole parent families live in poverty' (Morris and Trethewey 1988: 28). This situation is confirmed by Saunders (1994: 141). After showing that poverty increased over the 1980s for all of the family types he identified, Saunders (1994: 141) concludes:

The family types most at risk were sole parent families and, in 1989–90, single elderly people. For sole parent families, the poverty rates . . . are nothing short of alarming – around 44 per cent in 1981–2 and over 58 per cent in 1989–90.

Two other categories of people need also to be mentioned, in that although comparatively small in number, both reflect a very difficult and serious poverty situation. The population of homeless youth – youth separated from their families of origin and living virtually on the street – has been increasing in many countries, of which Australia is one. Yet they rarely figure in the general statistics because it represents a small and relatively invisible population. Hartley (1990) found many with incomes well below the poverty line, and among them pregnant women and former wards of state being in extreme need. Generally, however, the dimensions of this area of poverty are unknown; only its severity is beyond doubt.

The second category of people who represent a poverty situation of major concern are the Aboriginal population. As Pollard (1988: 9) has said, 'Aboriginal poverty is pervasive and intractable.' It is also extremely complex, not least because 'welfare dependency breeds problems beyond the poverty it meant to alleviate' (p. 9). Aboriginal poverty relates to very high levels of unemployment, to welfare dependency, to high levels of alcoholism and associated violence, to problems of articulating identity in a white society, to lack of self-esteem and a sense of not belonging, to early injustices and misguided policies, to persisting racism and discrimination – small wonder that Pollard (1988: 112) concludes: 'Aboriginal poverty remains one of the most perplexing and deep-seated difficulties in Australian social welfare today.'

Certainly it is not a poverty where income, or its absence, is either the major factor or the major measure.

Finally, in identifying categories of people in poverty some mention must be made of immigrants, especially newly-arrived immigrants. The Henderson Poverty Inquiry found that, as a disability group, recent immigrants had a poverty rate of only 2.6 per cent – just under the 2.7 per cent figure for those with no disability. When all migrant units were considered, however, the figure went to 9.8 per cent – very similar to the overall population figure of 10.2 per cent. However, 'the recent migrant group is the only one whose situation after housing deteriorates significantly', for it moved from 2.6 to 5.2 per cent, but was still below the overall figure of 6.7 per cent (Australia, Commission of Inquiry into Poverty 1975: 19).

What the Henderson Poverty Inquiry found, however, was that recent migrants frequently possessed what was termed 'multiple disabilities'. Of the 40,000 recent migrants with other disabilities,

28.8 per cent were 'very poor' before housing and 31.3 per cent after housing. The additional disabilities confronting recent migrants in poverty were single females with no children, unemployed, large families and aged. For example, '4.8 'per cent of all recent migrant adult income units had an 'unemployment' disability, compared with 1.6 per cent for all other income units' (Australia, Commission of Inquiry into Poverty 1975: 20).

Overall then, 'the incidence of poverty among newly-arrived migrants was nearly double that of the general population, after housing costs had been deducted' (Martin 1976: 182). As with the Aboriginal population, however, this was again a poverty situation of considerable complexity. Cultural backgrounds, adaptation to Australian services, inadequate services for recently-arrived migrants and other factors were all seen by the Henderson Poverty Inquiry as contributing to the above average poverty rate among immigrants in Australia.

In 1991 Johnson's report on poverty among immigrants was published. He discovered an alarming situation, namely that 'immigrant poverty increased by 48 per cent between 1981–2 and 1985–6, compared with an increase of 27 per cent in poverty among all Australians' (p. 34). Poverty was found to be particularly high among immigrants from a non-English-speaking background, and those with a secondary school education or less. It should be noted, however, that 'the level of poverty was much the same for immigrants as a whole and for Australian-born' (p. 26); the two key factors determining poverty were years of residence and language background. To be from a non-English-speaking background and to be recently arrived would dramatically increase the likelihood of poverty (pp. 30–3).

We can summarise the data available on the groups most affected by poverty in two ways. First, we can identify categories of persons at greatest risk: single-parent households, especially if female headed; the elderly, especially if living alone; the homeless youth population; and recently-arrived immigrants from a non-English-speaking background. Then, because of the strong family orientation in much of this listing, we can identify children as bearing the brunt of poverty far more than adults. Second, we can identify those most likely to be in poverty in terms of income source. Of course to do this is to focus exclusively on the income factor in poverty, yet without neglecting the non-income dimensions of poverty one would have to conclude that income has been and remains a crucial factor. Two major sources of income are involved – employment-generated income and social security pensions and benefits income. Clearly paid work is the best way to avoid poverty in Australia, yet the 1980s did see the growing importance of a new class of 'working poor' in Australia – those employed for short periods, part-time workers or with large families on low wages. Yet as Saunders (1994: 274) concludes: 'if a paid job does not always guarantee an income above the poverty line, not being in the labour force at all is associated with the highest overall risk of poverty'. The implication of this is that income security provisions in Australia will not always serve to keep people out of poverty.

Before closing this section on groups most affected by poverty it is important to consider the rural sector, although it is not an area frequently highlighted in Australia. The Henderson Poverty Inquiry did contract research into rural poverty, but found that the difficulty about making comparisons between farm and non-farm families is that there was a large number of rural income units with 'incomes obviously totally inadequate for them to live on', but 'low income among people who own and operate businesses is not a good indication of poverty' (Australia, Commission of Inquiry into Poverty 1975: 179).

The findings from these studies suggested that 'aged persons and sub-commercial farms accounted for a substantial proportion of those farmers at risk of poverty' (Australia, Commission of Inquiry into Povety 1975: 180). In addition, the large variability in farm income over the year was often a problem for farmers, so that variation from year to year in climatic and price factors meant that temporary poverty was a common feature of farm life. Finally, it was clear that there was also considerable variation between different types of farming and different farming areas.

The Henderson Poverty Inquiry found that 'of the 399,000 income units in Australia with incomes, before housing costs, less than the poverty line, 142,000 were living in rural areas' (Australia, Commission of Inquiry into Poverty 1975: 187). After housing costs that proportion dropped markedly, reflecting the lower cost of housing in rural areas. The higher incidence of poverty is due in part to two characteristics – a marginally higher proportion of the aged and a higher incidence of unemployment in rural areas. The dominant reason, however, was the low incomes of rural working people, especially rural labourers of whom 18.4 per cent were 'very poor' and 14.6 per cent were 'rather poor' before housing costs. A study of rural poverty over the 1968–9 to 1972–3 period by Vincent (quoted in Davidson and Lees 1993: 9) found that 'about 12 per cent of farm households had incomes below the poverty line', but went on to conclude, 'a closer investigation revealed that many small households comprised aged persons, operating small acreages, and producing little commercial output'.

Davidson and Lees (1993) found that rural poverty varied from 18 to 24 per cent, depending on the area. The highest incidence was among the unemployed, but 33 per cent of self-employed farmer households were found to be in poverty. They concluded from their findings that the 28 per cent rural poverty incidence, when compared to the 22 per cent national poverty incidence, was not excessive, given the rural recession at the time and the very different situation of rural families compared to urban families. And, as other studies have found, unemployment, dependence on social security, and disabilities (such as being elderly) contributed significantly to the incidence of rural poverty.

FACTORS CONTRIBUTING TO POVERTY IN AUSTRALIA

Employment status is clearly the key factor in poverty in Australia. The 1975 Henderson Poverty Inquiry emphasised that the single most important determinant of poverty in the 1970s was unemployment, yet, at that stage, the unemployment rate was around 2.5 per cent. Hence the high rates of unemployment of recent decades (9–10 per cent) have been a major factor in creating and maintaining poverty. Saunders (1994: 272), and most other commentators, reflect that the relationship between poverty and labour force status remains critical. Moreover, the growth of employment after 1983 was due in large part to an increase in the labour force participation of married women, and an increase in the prevalence of part-time work (from 16 per cent to over 21 per cent of all employment). Hence despite a growth in employment, 'the number of families with neither partner in employment continued to rise, both absolutely and as a percentage of all couples' (Saunders 1993: 40).

One reason for the central importance of the employment factor in the causation of poverty is that a wages policy has often substituted for social policy (Castles 1994: 8). The arbitrated wages policy was expected to keep people out of poverty, but this, of course, failed miserably as unemployment rates rose. Clearly, however, structural factors relating to employment were also important. The nature of employment growth in the 1980s meant that the number of two-income families increased, while the plight of less qualified one-income units and of youth grew worse. A much bigger proportion of the unemployed faced long-term unemployment than had ever been true in the past. In January 1990, for example, 26.1 per cent of the 550,400 persons with no paid employment had been in that situation for more than a year (Brotherhood of St Laurence 1990: 21), and this situation has been maintained. While unemployment has been a key factor in the causation of poverty, it was only one factor for it is apparent that even the boom employment years of the 1950s and 1960s did not end poverty. Indeed, during that boom period some 20 per cent of the population were left behind. We must, therefore, look beyond labour market participation for other key factors.

A second key poverty causation factor was the housing market. Australian social policy favoured private ownership of place of residence, and fiscal policy helped many to achieve this goal. As one outcome of this policy, however, public housing has always received a low priority, while the rental market was for many years left to market forces. Hence the Henderson Poverty Inquiry (Australia, Commission of Inquiry into Poverty 1975: 24) found

> that renters from private landlords are a group whose situation is worst after housing costs. They comprise only 21.4 per cent of all adult income units but constitute 40.8 per cent of adult income units below the poverty line on an after-housing basis.

In the mid-1980s, public housing lists were longer while public housing remained an area of low government priority, and according to Disney (1987: 2): 'the waiting lists for public housing have lengthened very considerably, while for many low income people private rental levels have increased sharply and housing loans have become more expensive.' The situation has not improved since.

A third key causal factor in poverty in Australia is educational attainment level. The 1975 Henderson Poverty Inquiry found that 'poverty does increase with a decreased amount of schooling' (Australia, Commission of Inquiry into Poverty 1975: 24). The situation identified in more recent studies is that the rate and duration of unemployment is closely related to educational attainment. Crossley (1990: 8) found that completing secondary school was a watershed. A poverty taskforce in Western Australia found that 'educational attainment is the most important factor in employment status' (WACOSS 1990: 4).

A fourth causal factor in poverty is Australia's distinctive non-contributory social assistance system. It cannot be ignored that many of those in poverty are social security recipients. The 1975 Henderson Poverty Inquiry (1975: 23) found that a poverty gap existed for all types of pensioner and beneficiary income units with no other income; and that

(i) single pensioners, with no children, and fatherless families are the ones worst off (i.e. with the highest poverty gap); (ii) large families (both intact and fatherless) are worse off than small families; (iii) married couples with no children are only just below the poverty line.

The Henderson Poverty Inquiry's (1975: 65) first recommendation in this area was, therefore, to raise pension rates to the poverty line, although it suggested a whole range of measures for improving the social assistance system.

Analysing the situation which prevailed during the 1980s, Saunders (1994: 26) found that the poverty rate amongst those receiving government income-support payments in both 1981–2 and 1989–90 was well above the national poverty rate. At the same time, there were also a considerable number of people in poverty who were not receiving any income-support payments from government. He concludes that Australia's categorical social assistance system is thus not very effectively targeted on the poor. At the same time he questions the assumption that the only goal of a social assistance system is poverty alleviation. Furthermore, Australia's publicly funded social assistance system is dependent on continued public support, and the increasing emphasis on targeting, Saunders (1994: 45) concludes, 'may well have undermined broad-based public support for social security and thus led to a lower level of social security expenditure'.

In this context it is important also to make reference to the creation of poverty traps by the interaction of the social assistance and taxation systems. When social assistance recipients earn above a set limit their pension or benefit is reduced and they may be taxed on their earnings. This discourages social assistance recipients from working and thus creates a poverty trap (ACTCOSS 1986: 39). There is often a dilemma in this area which relates to fears of welfare dependency. As Disney (1987: 6) expresses it: 'Increased social security is necessary but there can be no doubt that the greatest assistance for many people in hardship is to help them to provide largely for themselves rather than increase their long-term dependency on the State.'

While a logical and laudable argument, the dilemma is that Australian policy has always feared welfare dependency, but in recent decades it has also failed either to generate adequate employment opportunities or to identify alternative self-reliance strategies. Moreover, for various reasons the eligibility for social assistance has been radically tightened, while the average level of assistance provided relative to living costs has fallen.

Finally, it must be said that poverty in Australia is related to social exclusion. This is certainly the case with Aboriginal poverty, but is also apparent in relation to homeless youth and single older men with characteristics of destitution. It would also be true to say that both single-parent households and some recently-arrived immigrant populations have experienced a degree of animosity and discrimination. While there are signs, in both cases, that social exclusion is less in the mid-1990s than even a decade ago, it is still there to a sufficient degree to render life difficult for both populations. Finally, the experiences of state wards, those convicted of crimes and those committed to psychiatric institutions can find their efforts to avoid poverty somewhat frustrated. In each of these situations, the impact of one or more of the poverty causation factors is intensified to at least some degree by the factor of social exclusion.

THE SOCIAL WELFARE RESPONSES TO POVERTY IN AUSTRALIA

Australian responses to poverty have occurred at different levels. The central response which emerged early in Australia's history was premised on the idea that through employment and wages policies there would be no poverty. The prevailing public attitude was certainly that all men (and historically the emphasis was on men) should and needed to work. It was important to self-image and essential for supporting oneself and one's dependants. The two planks of this central economic approach were the provision of jobs and the establishment and maintenance of a minimum wage. Historically, as Jones (1990: 14–17) sees it, early in Australia's development 'the newly powerful working classes, through their political arm the Australian Labor Party, were interested in creating a protected "welfare state" for those on wages'. The Australian economy became 'one of the most heavily protected in the world' to protect jobs; while: 'The philosophy of wage control in the 1890s played a vital part in Australian social policy development, and Australian social policy has remained heavily dependent on wages and conditions regulations' (Jones 1990: 16).

Basic wage provisions were introduced in 1907, with the federal government having wide-ranging conciliation and arbitration powers from 1904. The first president of the Conciliation and Arbitration Court, Justice Higgins,

> listed thirty-three principles for the protection of the worker and talked of the role of wage regulations in giving 'immense relief to the thousands of helpless families', of lifting up the manhood of the poor, and for the proper sustenance for the upbringing of the children of a nation.
>
> (Jones 1990: 17)

As with all occupational welfare, the main danger with this approach was that it meant nothing for those not in the workforce. As Jones (1990: 14) comments, 'other workers had little interest in the poor removed from the workforce', and were disinclined to welcome taxes which would be used to fund social security provisions. However, the philosophy was that employment was the key to the resolution of poverty and the 1975 Henderson Poverty Inquiry found this still to be the situation at that time (1975: 128): 'The Commission found that there was widespread and strong belief in the desirability of men having a job and that employment was important for a person's self-image and his functioning as a member of a family and society.' The Henderson Poverty Inquiry stressed also the importance of ensuring that all employees came under the minimum wage award, noting that the extent of such coverage had been recently eroded. It commented (1975: 130): 'By raising minimum wages steadily over many years the Arbitration Commission has undoubtedly made a major contribution to the reduction of poverty among those at work.'

The Henderson Poverty Inquiry (1975: 132), of course, noted that the prevailing incidence of poverty had much to do with the rate of unemployment, but it also noted that 'community attitudes to those out of work are often both negative and based on ignorance and suspicion'. The implication was that to use strategies other than employment-generation and minimum wages would not be very popular, and might therefore be politically unpalatable.

In any event, it has become increasingly apparent that an employment wages response to poverty is not effective. The government's capacity to ensure full employment through economic management is limited; the capacity of workers and others to ensure an appropriate minimum wage for all is equally limited, having declined steadily since the 1970s; and the phenomenon of the male as the sole income-earner in every family belongs to the past. Australia's key response to poverty has thus been significantly eroded since the 1970s; and in any case it offered no protection in periods such as the great depression of the 1930s. Yet employment policy has continued to be a major strategy in combating poverty, although, as Pollard (1992: 71) states:

> The emphasis is now on targeting specific unemployed groups as they are identified, with the aim of keeping them off welfare, minimising welfare dependency, and reinforcing the value of employment as the normal and natural means of meeting human needs.

This brings us to the second element in Australia's response to poverty, namely a social assistance response. Australia started to introduce social assistance pensions and benefits towards the end of the nineteenth century. The system that emerged was 'a single-tier formal social welfare system where benefits were flat rate, regardless of previous earnings, and were payable without contributions' (Jones 1990: 32). Behind the system was 'a view of government as a source of a minimum standard below which vulnerable groups should not fall' (Jones 1990: 356). 'These early pensions set the pattern for the later development of the Australian welfare state' (Jones 1990: 21).

Social assistance has broadened its coverage over the years. In 1899 the first age pension was introduced and a national scheme established in 1909. Invalid pensions were introduced in 1909. Family allowance, widow's pension and unemployment and special benefits followed in the 1941–5 period. In the 1970s the social security needs of the single-parent household were recognised, with the introduction of a Supporting Parents Benefit, first for females and then for males. In the 1980s a family income allowance as a further protection against family poverty was introduced.

While Australia's social assistance scheme has in recent decades broadened in coverage, it has at the same time narrowed its eligibility through tighter means testing and more poverty targeting of beneficiary categories. This process of assessing eligibility inevitably results in some persons and families losing their protection against poverty. For example, until June 1991 all Australian residents were entitled to non-contributory, means-tested unemployment benefits as a right for an indefinite period. A new policy introduced in 1991 turned unemployment benefits into training or job search allowances with a concern to prevent people 'choosing to refrain from entering the workforce' (Pollard 1992: 64). A subsequent policy change was to force adolescents to remain dependent on their parents, thus pushing some who chose to live independently into poverty. Policies designed largely to encourage people to return to work, or to living with parents, will inevitably result in poverty in certain circumstances. A final example, which has brought much protest, was the decision that from June 1996 Family Allowance for a child should cut out at age 16, although students can obtain a means-tested Basic Student Payment. The fear is that this will result frequently in a suspension of education, which in turn may jeopardise future employment because of the shortage of work for the unqualified.

If the coverage of social assistance was a major concern from the 1970s, so too were the levels of pensions and benefits. The 1975 Henderson Poverty Inquiry highlights the plight of pensioners and beneficiaries with no other income, and its proposal of a guaranteed minimum income made a lot of sense. Yet, as Saunders (1994: 23) points out, 'this proposal received only luke-warm support at the time and the general principle probably has even less support now'. The preferred alternative has always been the 'categorical approach', despite the fact, as Saunders (1994: 26) comments, that 'a categorical social security system is not very effectively targeted on the poor'. While the arguments for and against the Australian approach may be complex, the undeniable reality is that Australia's social assistance system as a response to poverty has not been very effective in the past and still is not.

The third response to poverty in Australia is charity, which is important because of its social significance over a long period. Australia has a long history of charitable institutions, many of which arrived from England in colonial days. In the nineteenth century institutional care prevailed. For example, in the State of Victoria in 1888–9 a total of 3 per cent of the population spent some time in one of its many institutions (Jones 1990: 20). By the 1930s that situation was paralleled by a large network of community-based relief organisations. In the 1980s and 1990s, as deinstitutionalisation led to the closure of most institutions, the community-relief response has been dominated by the non-government, non-profit welfare centres, which provide free or cheap clothing and furniture, food packages, overnight or short-term accommodation, and monetary gifts or loans.

In the 1990s, the volume of charitable relief has grown enormously, placing considerable strain on the distributing agencies and indirectly exerting considerable pressure on government to increase its welfare effort. Temporary accommodation facilities have been in very high demand, indicating the large numbers and increased range of homeless. Even more serious has been the level of demand from families for relief, reflecting large-scale temporary unemployment as well as the more entrenched problem situations.

There are many difficulties with the charitable response to poverty. Fundamentally it offers no more than a temporary respite, although in many agencies relief is complemented by other services designed to assist a family or person to become independent again. Second, the availability of such relief is very uneven, both geographically and temporally. Third, the process is, for many clients, a demeaning one. Accordingly, many will access it only if they are really desperate. A final problem is that such relief deters governments from adopting better and more broadly based programmes that will provide adequate income-support in the face of poverty or, preferably, its eradication.

The fourth response is a somewhat more nebulous grouping of discrete policy strategies that impact directly or indirectly on poverty. Fiscal policies have sought, successfully on the whole, to bring about a high level of home ownership. That level of ownership, especially once the house is free of debt, has buttressed many people against poverty, in that the cost of housing for non-owners has been a major factor in pushing people into poverty. Child-care policies have sought to satisfy an essential requirement of women re-entering the workforce. Although the provision of child-care has, unfortunately, a chequered history in Australia, where it has been available it has proved to be an important factor in mitigating poverty. Legal aid policy is another example, for many studies have shown how the high cost of justice has either deprived poor people of it or has rendered them destitute in its pursuit.

While all of the above poverty responses, together with a range of other services, have constituted individually and collectively a barrier to poverty, and sometimes even a remedy, the unfortunate reality is that poverty persists despite these measures. Private housing in Australia has become increasingly more expensive in recent times, while public housing remains the low priority that it has always been. Child-care facilities are not well subsidised, so that available places are often expensive and predominantly taken by the two-income families. Legal aid has been hard hit in recent times by government budget cuts, but the cost of litigation remains high. We must therefore conclude that these responses have never been specifically geared to the alleviation of poverty; and their ability to alleviate poverty is now far less than it was in the past.

The response to poverty among the Aboriginal people needs to be discussed separately. After an initial period of despicable treatment, government reserves were established to protect Aboriginal peoples against white settlers. Reserves reduced the people to virtually total dependency. With the gradual closure of the reserves, some recognition of land rights and a general increase in levels of white understanding, more power was devolved to Aboriginal communities in the 1970s. It is clearly impossible to respond to Aboriginal poverty using strategies appropriate to the rest of society. By and large employment opportunities are still barred by widespread discrimination, while government-funded self-help employment ventures have had mixed success. The social service response is a common one, but when it constitutes the only response its impact on self-esteem and sense of identity result in problems of alcoholism, violence, and high levels of disease and child neglect. A further response has been the establishment of Aboriginal services – housing, health, education and legal, for example – but these have been available from relatively few centres, rendering access a problem, and relatively poorly resourced. Many agree with Pollard (1988: 116) that community development is the only real alternative available, but that Aboriginal people will only develop as a community as they work on their own problems.

ANTI-POVERTY PROGRAMMES IN AUSTRALIA

At the preventive level, the use of employment and wage policies represent, in a sense, an anti-poverty programme if these can be implemented successfully. The possession of regular employment, together with the various components of occupational welfare (Bryson 1992: 131–42), is for many undoubtedly the best protection against poverty. However, the maintenance of full employment is only one among several competing economic policy objectives sought by recent Australian governments. Their capacity to maintain full employment, even when they choose to do so, would seem, however, to be limited. Moreover, there will always be a section of the population for whom entering the workforce is not a real option. It is not, therefore, sufficient to regard employment and wages policy as constituting a preventive anti-poverty programme, as some have been tempted to do (Pollard 1992). There are also many who question whether the advancement of the poor can take place through the operation of the welfare state. The Henderson Poverty Inquiry (1975: 3) concluded: 'Australia in the 1980s was going to be a hard country for the disadvantaged: there are going to be many people needing help and it is going to be more difficult to provide adequate welfare and community services.' This has proved to be all too accurate a prophecy. Inequality has grown considerably, and with it an increase in both relative and probably absolute poverty (Saunders 1994).

It could, therefore, be concluded that nowhere within Australia's responses to poverty can an anti-poverty programme as such be identified. Indeed, one might go further and argue that few in Australia would have ever seen the need for such a strategy. Prevailing attitudes towards the 'down-and-outers' (mainly homeless single males), the 'Aboriginal problem' and 'dole-bludgers' (those who preferred government support to being employed) were such that an anti-poverty programme does not constitute a politically viable response. Deterrent measures, such as maintaining low levels of social assistance pensions and benefits to encourage a return to the workforce, or training and other measures geared to ensuring a re-entry to the workforce were far more prevalent responses; although the latter have never targeted poverty while the former were never likely to have any impact on poverty.

THE LIKELIHOOD OF POVERTY IN AUSTRALIA IN THE FUTURE

So what of the future? Pollard (1992: 64) somewhat reluctantly suggests that there is an underclass in Australia:

> To the extent that there is an underclass in this country, it is composed of the long-term unemployed, the welfare dependent, alcoholics, drug abusers, homeless youth, and other groups outside mainstream cultural values or life styles. To a large extent these people are forced to have shortened perspectives, to focus on daily existence, and thereby become incapable of making long-term plans for their security.

Given this situation and that of the Aboriginal population, along with the lack of an anti-poverty programme, it would seem that in the future we shall witness a significant proportion of the Australian population living in poverty, although no projections are available.

For more than ten years now writers have been referring to 'the retreat from the welfare state', so that 'the position of the poorest and most vulnerable has deteriorated markedly' (Graycar 1983: 3). Writing more recently, Bryson (1992: 227) concludes that 'the limits of welfare state development have been reached, temporarily at least', and that the impact of the 'crisis of the welfare state' has fallen mainly on the poor. She elaborates (1992: 229–30):

> The benefits and advantages of the better-off have largely been maintained and even enhanced. Most of the belt-tightening has been done by those who are at the bottom of the social hierarchy . . . . The gap between rich and poor is widening . . . . The most vulnerable welfare state provisions are those targeted to subordinate groups which do not have the weight of middle-class support behind them.

Are there then no strategies available for tackling poverty in the future? Pollard (1992: 76) sees some hope in a community-based anti-poverty strategy:

> [t]he forces in modern western democracies making for individu-alism (or atomism or marginalism) are very strong and need to be

counterbalanced by forces which band individuals into communities and communities into commonwealths. Community development, as both process and outcome, has considerable potential to provide such a counterbalancing power.

Pollard, in distinguishing between community development in its Third World context and in the context of a high-income country, indicates (1992: 77) that 'In the latter, community development aims to incorporate marginalised groups of people into a social mainstream'.

Can a community development approach have a positive impact on poverty in Australia? If the experience to date is considered – Aboriginal community enterprises; workers taking over threatened enterprises in rural centres; ethnic groups' encouraging entrepreneurial activities; some indications of a western-style informal economy in the suburbs; and the construction of community facilities for leisure, and adult education – some optimism about the potential contribution of community development might be justified. Whether it is sufficient to eradicate poverty is, however, doubtful.

REFERENCES

Australian Capital Territory Council of Social Services (ACTCOSS) (1986) *Let Them Eat Cake . . . A Profile of Poverty in Canberra*, Canberra: ACTCOSS.

Australia, Commission of Inquiry into Poverty (1975) *Poverty in Australia: First Main Report*, Canberra: Australian Government Printing Service.

Australian Council of Social Services (ACOSS) (1988) *Keeping the Promise: A Strategy for Reducing Child Poverty*, Sydney: Australian Council of Social Service.

Brotherhood of St Laurence (BSL) (1990) *Australians in Poverty: A Resource Book*, Melbourne: Brotherhood of St Laurence.

Bryson, L. (1992) *Welfare and the State*, London, Macmillan.

Carter, J. (ed.) (1991) *Measuring Child Poverty: Child Poverty Review*, Melbourne: Brotherhood of St Laurence.

Castles, F.G. (1994) *The Wage Earners Welfare State Revisited: Refurbishing the Established Model of Social Protection* (Discussion Paper No. 39), Canberra: Australian National University Graduate Program in Public Policy.

Choo, C. (1990) *Aboriginal Child Poverty*, Melbourne: Brotherhood of St Laurence.

Crossley, L. (1990) *Children and the Future of Work*, Melbourne: Brotherhood of St Laurence.

Davidson, B. and Lees, J. (1993) *An Investigation of Poverty in Rural and Remote Regions of Australia*, Armidale, NSW: Rural Development Centre, University of New England.

Disney, J. (1987) *Poverty, Wealth and Public Welfare*, Sydney: Australian Council of Social Service.

Graycar, A. (ed.) (1983) *Retreat from the Welfare State: Australian Social Policy in the 1980s*, Sydney: Allen and Unwin.

Graycar, A. and Jamrozik, A. (1993) *How Australians Live: Social Policy in Theory and Practice* (2nd edn), Sydney: Macmillan.

Harris, P. (1989) *Child Poverty, Inequality and Social Justice*, Melbourne: Brotherhood of St Laurence.

Hartley, R. (1990) *What Price Independence? Report of a Study of Young People's Incomes and Living Costs*, Melbourne: Youth Affairs Council of Australia.

Henderson, R.F., Harcourt, A. and Harper, R.J.A. (1970) *People in Poverty, A Melbourne Survey*, Melbourne: Cheshire.

Henderson R.F. (1981) *The Welfare Stakes: Strategies for Australian Social Policy*, Melbourne: Institute of Applied Economic and Social Research, University of Melbourne.

Hollingworth, P. (1972) *The Powerless Poor. A Comprehensive Guide to Poverty in Australia*, Melbourne: Stockland Press.

Johnson, D. (1991) *The Measurement and Extent of Poverty Among Immigrants*, Canberra: Australian Government Printing Service.

Johnson, D., Manning, I. and Hellwig, O. (1995) *Trends in the Distribution of Cash Income and Non-Cash Benefits* (Report to the Department of the Prime Minister and Cabinet), Canberra: Australian Government Publishing Service.

Jones, M.A. (1990) *The Australian Welfare State: Origins, Control and Choices*, (3rd edn), Sydney, Allen and Unwin.

McCaughey, J. (1987) *A Bit of a Struggle: Coping with Family Life in Australia*, Melbourne: Penguin Books.

Martin, G.S. (1976) *Social/Medical Aspects of Poverty in Australia* (Third Main Report), Canberra: Australian Government Printing Service for the Australian Government Commission of Inquiry into Poverty.

Morris, H. and Trethewey, J. (1988) *Sole Parents and the 1987 Amendments to the Social Security Act*, Melbourne: Brotherhood of St Laurence.

Pollard, D. (1988) *Give and Take: The Losing Partnership in Aboriginal Poverty*, Sydney: Hale and Iremonger.

—— (1992) *Social Need and Social Policy: The Economic Content of Social Welfare*, Sydney: Hale and Iremonger.

Saunders, P. (1992) *Longer Run Changes in the Distribution of Income in Australia*, Sydney: Social Policy Research Centre, University of New South Wales.

—— (1993) *Economic Adjustment and Distributional Change: Income Inequality in Australia in the 1980s*, Sydney: Social Policy Research Centre, University of New South Wales.

—— (1994) *Welfare and Inequality: National and International Perspectives on the Australian Welfare State*, Melbourne, Cambridge University Press.

Taylor, J. and McClelland, A. (1994) *Poverty and Inequality: A Welfare Organisation's Perspective*, Melbourne: Brotherhood of St Laurence.

Ternowetsky, G.W. (1980) *Intergenerational Poverty: Life Styles and Income Maintenance*, Canberra: Australian Government Printing Service.

Western Australian Council of Social Services (WACOSS) (1990) *Report on the Western Australian Poverty Taskforce*, Perth: WACOSS.

Chapter 3

Canada

Hugh Shewell

Canada! For many people, including a substantial number of Canadians, the name evokes a land of milk and honey, a land full of limitless opportunity for individuals willing and able to work hard. For them, to be poor in Canada is either unimaginable or the result of indolent, spendthrift or immoral behaviour. In a materially rich country, poverty is seen as a condition that can be avoided. Even conceding the existence of the poor, the generosity of the Canadian social safety net has, arguably, alleviated absolute poverty to such an extent that, by stark comparison to anywhere else in the world, the poor can hardly claim to be poor at all (Sarlo 1994). These laudatory images are however, quite misleading; for, as Canada's social safety net has been methodically dismantled in recent years, the reality of poverty worsens.

THE LAND AND ITS GOVERNMENT

Canada is an enormous, geographically diverse country occupying nearly 10 million square kilometres of the northern half of North America. Bordered by the Arctic, Atlantic and Pacific Oceans, and on the south by the United States of America, it is dominated by the Canadian Shield, a rugged, largely infertile upland, rich in mineral deposits. The Maritime provinces, southern Québec and Ontario however, are characterised by rolling landscapes and are suitable for mixed agricultural production. The fertile, central plains are famous for their wheat production. In the west, the land is mountainous and richly forested from the Rockies through to the Pacific coastal ranges.

While agriculture, fishing, forestry and mining have remained important since the Second World War, Canada has also become a major, industrial power. More recently the emergence of viable service industries have propelled the nation towards a post-industrial economic structure. Although primary industry is fairly evenly distributed over the country, secondary industry is located mainly in southern Ontario and Québec.

Globalisation and the implementation of free trade with the United States (1988) – expanded to Mexico under the North American Free Trade Agreement (1994) – caused a significant restructuring of Canada's economy and labour force the effects of which were felt primarily in Ontario and Québec. Hundreds of thousands of jobs were lost when industries either relocated to lower wage countries or simply shut down (Barlow and Campbell 1995; Watkins 1992; Teeple 1995). New industries are gradually replacing those lost, but many of them are either in less labour intensive and in high technology and related fields, or in insecure, low-paying service sector areas such as sales and fast foods. The new industrial structure is also creating a dual economy with a resultant polarisation of income: high-technology and goods-producing industries employ relatively few at high wages while the service sector employs many more at very low wages. In the meantime there is a continuing decline in the middle income group (Ternowetsky and Riches 1993: 11–16). These developments have also been paralleled by Canada's gradual abandonment of Keynesian economic intervention strategies, the welfare state, and the implicit surrender of its own sense of economic and, to some extent, political sovereignty (Barlow 1996; Barlow and Campbell 1995; Laxer 1995; Shields and McBride 1994; Scott 1996; Teeple 1995; Ternowetsky and Riches 1993; Watkins 1992).

Canada is a federal, parliamentary democracy consisting of ten provinces and two territories. The federal parliament is in Ottawa, while each province has its own capital and legislature. The Yukon and the Northwest Territories are still under the authority of Ottawa which delegates power to their respective legislatures. Each government has a complex public administration to implement the legislation, policies and on-going business of the state. Ottawa and the provinces derive their jurisdictional powers from the constitution, originally named the British North America Act (1867), now the Constitution Act (1982).

The division of powers is crucial to understanding Canada's inability to develop comprehensive, enduring strategies to combat poverty. Section 91 of the Constitution, which specifies the federal powers, is considered to take precedence over Section 92, which specifies the provincial powers. In addition however, Sections 102 and 106 enable the federal government to create a consolidated revenue fund and to spend money from that fund 'for the Public Service' meaning, in effect, for the public good or interest. The combination of these two powers is referred to as the federal spending power by which Ottawa has invoked the use of conditional grants to the provinces (Irving 1987). Why is this important? First, under Section 92 the provincial governments have sole jurisdiction of social welfare, as well as of civil rights and property including insurance. Under Section 91, the federal government has by far the greatest power to raise taxes both directly and indirectly. Historically, the provinces have been unable to sustain the funding of social welfare programmes without federal help, yet constitutionally the federal government does not have the authority to enter into what is provincial jurisdiction. When, in Canada's early history, the federal government tried to enter areas of provincial jurisdiction using its general power to maintain peace and order it was overruled by the British Judicial Committee of the Privy Council (Irving 1987). There are only three ways around the dilemma: use constitutional amendments to give the federal government specific powers in an area of provincial jurisdiction (for example, Unemployment Insurance); use federal spending powers in ways that do not legally infringe on provincial jurisdiction; or rely on the provinces to finance their own programmes (Guest 1985).

The advantages of the first two methods are threefold. First, a strong federal presence in social welfare promotes national unity and a sense of community. Second, the federal government, by using its spending power and the conditional grant, can set national social welfare programme standards and cost share with the provinces, providing they adhere to these standards which ensure that citizens, regardless of where they live in Canada, receive reasonably comparable levels of social security and equitable treatment. Finally, federal involvement in social welfare contributes to a greater sense of equality among the provinces and helps to decrease perceptions of regional disparity. Indeed, the use of the federal spending power in the form of transfer payments to the provinces is one way in which Canada can combat poverty at a macro socio-economic level.

The disadvantages have been recently resurrected and spring from the wealth of some provinces coupled with a strong ideological movement to the right. These provinces – especially Alberta and

Ontario – see the use of the federal spending power as an intrusion on their powers and a barrier to their ideological goal to minimise the role of the state in social welfare. Consequently, they and Québec – which for other political and cultural reasons opposes the federal presence in social welfare – have been agitating for a greatly reduced federal presence in social welfare. Although this position is more in keeping with the original intent of the Constitution, it has been shown repeatedly over time to be fiscally problematic for the provinces, especially the poorer ones. While it may satisfy the urge of the richer provinces to exert their independence in the confederation, it would – in the opinion of many observers – lead to a fragmented, regionally disparate social welfare system and, therefore, a country of radically unequal citizenship (Moscovitch 1996; Riches 1997; Silver 1996).

THE PEOPLE: SOME DEMOGRAPHIC CHARACTERISTICS

Canada today is a nation of about thirty million people. At the time of confederation in 1867, it was composed primarily of its aboriginal inhabitants (that is, North American Indians, the Métis – persons of mixed European and Indian ancestry – and the Inuit), and persons of either British or French origin. Since 1867, through successive waves of immigration, Canada's demography has changed significantly. For the next hundred years immigrants were drawn mainly from continental Europe, the United Kingdom, Ireland and the United States. Persons of non-European origin were mainly excluded (McNaught 1988; Morton 1983). In the past thirty years however, immigration has come increasingly from the developing countries and the Asia-Pacific. Between 1981 and 1991 Europeans accounted for 25 per cent of Canada's immigrants, a decline of 65 per cent since 1961. In contrast, between 1981 and 1991 of the 1.2 million immigrants to Canada, 50 per cent were from Asia and the Middle East, while an additional 20 per cent came from Africa, South America and the Caribbean. By 1991, 16 per cent of Canada's population was directly immigrant in origin. While 54 per cent were still European by birth, fully 40 per cent were born in Asia, the Middle East, Africa, South and Central America and the Caribbean (Badets 1994).

In 1867 Canada was an agricultural, pre-industrial society. Only three cities had populations over 30,000 and 80 per cent of the population was rural (Guest 1985). In the late 1980s this is reversed: only 20 per cent of the population live in rural areas (Biggs and Bollman 1994). Nine cities have metropolitan populations in excess of half a million while four of these exceed one million. Toronto, the largest, is over four million (Statistics Canada 1996).

Canada has an ageing population. Following the post Second World War baby boom the Canadian median age dropped to a low of 25.4 years, but since 1970 it has steadily risen to a high in 1992 of 33.8 years. This trend will continue unless there is a significant change in the natural birth rate and/or the rate of immigration is increased (McKie 1994).

The average income for all Canadian households in 1994 was C\$45,190; the median income, C\$37,730. The average and median family incomes in the same year were considerably higher than this (C\$55,080 and C\$48,970 respectively), while average and median incomes for unattached persons were similarly lower (C\$23,820 and C\$18,100) (Ross, Shillington and Lochhead 1994).

Canada's labour force grew steadily beginning in the late 1960s, but by 1989 this growth had slowed considerably and the average age of the labour force had begun to rise. A significant factor in the growth was the entry of the post-war generation into the labour market. Most importantly, women's participation in the labour force rose steadily from 38 per cent in 1969 to 58 per cent by 1989, while men's participation declined one percentage point over the same period, from 78 to 77 per cent. The unemployment rate rose steadily during the 1970s, stabilised, then rose sharply again during the recession of the 1980s. Although it declined from a peak of 11.8 per cent in 1983 it remains unacceptably high at over 9 per cent in 1996 (Parliament 1994; *The Globe and Mail* (Toronto) 12 October 1996). It is also generally conceded that actual unemployment is higher since the official rate does not count those on basic social assistance nor those who, out of despair of finding work, have dropped out of the labour market. Finally, the distribution of occupational groups in Canada has changed greatly since 1911. In that year, agriculture accounted for 34 per cent of all occupations, but by 1986 it accounted for only 4 per cent. Also, in 1911, 8 per cent of occupations were evenly distributed among clerical and professional groupings but by 1986 this had risen to 35 per cent of which clerical occupations accounted for 19 per cent. While manufacturing, transport, construction, and primary industries have retained a relatively consistent share of occupational distribution (39 per cent in 1911, 37 per cent in 1986), commercial/financial and service sector occupations have risen 9 per cent since 1911 to 24 per cent in 1986 (O'Neill 1994). Overall, there has been a significant decline in occupations dependent mainly on physical labour and a rise in those dependent on higher education and/or the acquisition of specialised, technical skills.

THE HISTORICAL AND POLITICAL CONTEXT OF POVERTY

Canada was born of political and economic expedience to advance British North American business interests and to protect them from the rapacious American commerce and culture to the south. There was no popular demand for independence from Britain. Rather, a powerful, mainly English-speaking elite residing in central Canada saw the need for greater independence from London in order to enhance both their and the overall interests of the British Empire (Naylor 1987). A nation-state in the mould of those created elsewhere in the mid-nineteenth century, was constituted specifically to protect property and to advance capitalist interests (Hobsbawm 1990; MacPherson 1977). Indeed, there was nothing very democratic about Canada at its inception; aboriginal peoples, the working class – such as it was – and women were accorded few rights. They were either not of or were mere appendages to society. In this sense the history of poverty and the struggle for social change and social justice in Canada are mainly the history and struggle of the working class, of women and of aboriginal peoples.

The constitutional division of powers reflect the nineteenth century understanding of, and importance attached to, poverty and social welfare; they were matters of a local or private nature, to be dealt with as provincial or municipal authorities saw fit (Guest 1985). The great powers of state were given to the federal government, while those considered to be associated with the routine administration of daily affairs were accorded to the provinces. Because of Canada's early agrarian base, there was no thought given to poverty of the kind spawned by urban industrialisation nor of its potential ramifications upon the interests of state and capital (Guest 1985; Irving 1987).

Constitutionally, then, Ottawa had no inherent interest in the existence of poverty *per se*, while the provinces, although they had the power, were disinclined to involve the state in matters which could be dealt with by residual, charitable means (Guest 1985; Irving 1987). Only when poverty became an issue of staggering proportions during the Great Depression of the 1930s was the Constitution found wanting, both in the division of powers and in the related fiscal capability of the provinces to intervene. In Canada's first quarter century, then, poverty was not perceived by the state to be a major public issue. Beginning with Canada's industrialisation in the 1890s, however, and through to the aftermath of the First World War both the incidence of, and public and state perceptions of poverty and its causes began to change (Guest 1985; Moscovitch and Drover 1987).

Industrialisation, as it did elsewhere, caused a significant movement of the population to urban areas. Directly and indirectly it produced over-crowded and inadequate housing, poor sanitation, unsafe working conditions, low wages, child labour, increased crime, family problems, alcoholism; in short, the conditions and behaviours associated with poverty and oppression. Among the organised responses to these conditions were coalitions of labour, women's temperance unions, left-wing political parties, and Christian social gospel movements which all held large rallies and conferences calling for social reform (Cook 1985; Guest 1985; Prentice *et al.* 1988).

During this early period of industrialisation attempts were also made to define and measure poverty. For the first time it began to be understood as a general and shared condition which transcended the supposed moral turpitude or laziness of those whom it most afflicted (Guest 1985). Two groups were seen to be most affected by poverty. The first, workers, had few rights, could not *effectively* unionise or strike, and worked in appalling conditions (Copp 1974; Guest 1985). There were no medical benefits, unemployment insurance, or employment standards to protect wages during illness: a sick or injured worker received no income and could lose his job. When injured workers began to sue factory owners for loss of livelihood, provincial governments in Ontario and Québec, together with the interested owners of big business, responded by introducing Workmen's Compensation benefits by which workers received a small income for lost wages but forfeited the right to sue (Guest 1985). This was the first form of institutionalised state intervention in Canada to alleviate poverty. However, other popular demands for broader forms of social security and unemployment insurance were essentially ignored by the state (Guest 1985).

A second group severely affected by industrialisation were persons forced to retire for reasons of age. In effect, the state did not distinguish between any class of worker who had become non-productive. Thus, retired workers were simply abandoned by employers and the state after years of working for poor wages. Again, popular calls for old age pensions were ignored. Instead, the federal and provincial response to poverty in old age was to encourage workers to save for their retirement, a nonsensical proposition when wages were inadequate in the first place (Guest 1985).

Towards the end of the First World War the state response to poverty began to change in small yet significant ways. This was due in part to the profound disillusion citizens felt towards the state following the senseless carnage of the war, and to the bourgeois fear of a communist revolution. The first change came in the form of pensions for returning veterans. This represented an important state recognition of their contribution to 'God and Country'. Their provision, however, revealed another problem. During the war, women were widowed in large numbers and, after the war, were displaced from their employment by men. As a result destitution among single-mothers rose dramatically. Provincial governments reluctantly acceded to the demands of women's and other organisations for a monthly, state income. Beginning in 1916, needs tested Mothers' Pensions were available in five provinces by 1920 (Guest 1985; Moscovitch and Drover 1987). A second post-war state response to poverty was an effort to combat unemployment and labour unrest. The federal government provided conditional grants to the provinces to establish employment brokerage offices. For a limited time, it also provided funds to the provinces for the provision of direct income relief and the initiation of public works (Guest 1985; Irving 1987).

A third, and final, state concession to poverty during this period was in 1927. The federal Liberal government of Mackenzie King, bowed to popular opinion and to the pressure of a small but formidable group of left-wing Members of Parliament, and passed the Old Age Pensions Act. Under this Act the federal government agreed to pay 50 per cent of the costs of provincially administered pensions to persons 70 years of age or over who qualified under a means test. It was the first, significant, federal presence in an area of social welfare on a continuing, non-emergency basis (Guest 1985).

The Great Depression of the 1930s revealed the true extent of Canada's inability to prevent or alleviate poverty. The fragile economy collapsed causing consistent unemployment levels above 20 per cent. Added to this was the onset of a harsh prairie drought occasioning destitution among farmers, and the bankruptcy of many municipalities. Finally, the laissez-faire dogma of the federal Conservative government of R.B. Bennett and its utter refusal to take meaningful action to ease the human distress only exacerbated the calamity (Finkel 1977; Guest 1985; Struthers 1983).

Fearing the destabilisation of capitalism and conscious of the growing popularity of left-wing parties in Canada a new, federal Liberal government initiated a Royal Commission to review the status of federal–provincial relations, to seek new fiscal arrangements, and to examine the future role of central government in the Canadian state. The report of this commission, known as the Rowell-Sirois Commission (1937–40), had the effect of dramatically altering the role and influence of the federal government in Canada. While many of its recommendations were rejected by the provinces, a more proactive role of the federal government gained popular favour. Thus, the Liberal government of Mackenzie King incrementally adopted several areas of its recommendations. These included a greater federal presence in national social security and the use of equalisation payments to the provinces (Guest 1985; Owram 1986; Simeon and Robinson 1990).

In 1940, as the economy gained strength due to the increased demands of the Second World War, the federal government implemented an unemployment insurance programme by obtaining a constitutional amendment giving it exclusive jurisdiction in that area. Then, between 1944 and 1954, following the *Report on Social Security for Canada* (1943), the federal government launched several socio-economic initiatives. The most important of these was a universal Family Allowance in 1944 and, in 1951, an enhanced, federally financed *and* administered, universal Old Age Pension. The former was accomplished through the use of the general spending power, while the latter required a further constitutional amendment (Guest 1985; Irving 1987). In the ensuing years up to 1966, Canada assembled the basic framework of a liberal, welfare state which included: an improved universal Old Age Pension, a contributory, employment-based pension plan, a cost-sharing plan with the provinces for a range of social and income services accompanied by national standards, and – perhaps the jewel in the crown

– a universally accessible, portable health care plan (Guest 1985; Moscovitch and Drover 1987). The international energy crisis of 1973 heralded the end of positive state welfare in Canada. The business community which benefited greatly from the social stability brought about by Canada's modest welfare state, was nevertheless ideologically opposed to state social spending (Haddow 1993). Throughout the 1980s this opposition became more intense as government deficits – and thus debts – increased. Liberal and Conservative federal governments – both of which uphold the primacy and preferability of private enterprise – were fairly easily convinced of the merit of resisting the further expansion of social programmes or of gradually eliminating them. Since the late 1970s both the federal and provincial governments have been in a gradual process of re-structuring Canada's social security. With the General Agreement on Tariffs and Trade, free trade and the globalisation of capital, the Canadian state, fully supported by the private sector, appears less interested in social rights of citizenship than in ensuring both a level economic playing field with the United States and Mexico, and an internationally competitive labour market (Geller and Joel 1996; Riches 1997: 65–9). The will to alleviate and minimise poverty through state intervention has been largely abandoned in favour of invoking the invisible hand of Adam Smith to create such enormous amounts of wealth through the marketplace that theoretically all will benefit.

Currently much of what Canadians have come to expect in social security has been eroded. Unemployment Insurance, re-named Employment Insurance, has been fundamentally restructured. The federal government no longer contributes to it but, as its regulator, has reduced the amount and length of benefits and made eligibility much more difficult. The Family Allowance has been eliminated in favour of tax targeting those 'most in need', while a similar fate has befallen the Old Age Pension. The future ability of the Canada Pension Plan to meet the needs of an ageing population remains in doubt and the health care system is under considerable pressure to become a two-tiered model favouring those who could afford a higher quality of care (Pulkingham and Ternowetsky 1996; Schellenberg 1996; Silver 1996).

Finally, beginning in the 1990s the federal government began to reduce the amounts transferred to the provinces for basic social assistance and personal social services. This action culminated in 1996 with a new block grant, the Canada Health and Social

Transfer (CHST) programme. Under CHST the federal government has terminated the national standards for social programmes articulated under the old plan. Instead, a new statement of principles and objectives are to be developed in consultation with the provinces. To date this has not been accomplished and some believe social welfare will return to its pre-Second World War format: a patchwork of highly selective, poorly funded, ideologically driven services (Moscovitch 1996; National Council of Welfare 1995; Pulkingham and Ternowetsky 1996).

Canada's efforts towards building a welfare state were mediocre and never approached the comprehensiveness of social democratic models found in Sweden and elsewhere. Rather, the Canadian model remained firmly in the liberal residual matrix, attaching the greatest benefits to employment-related activity (Myles 1988; Haddow 1993). Consequently, poverty was never substantially reduced and welfare state measures were only mildly redistributive. Still, it could be argued that the programmes that were in place minimised the worsening of poverty and pointed the way to its further alleviation. With their demise the future of social welfare and the implications for the incidence of poverty are bleak (Banting 1987; Battle 1994; Riches 1997).

POVERTY: THE PROBLEM OF AN APPROPRIATE DEFINITION

One of the continuing difficulties in any discussion about poverty is the question of definition. While the question has generally been a useful one among social scientists, in the past decade or so it has led to increasingly neo-liberal arguments about the extent to which poverty as a condition exists in the more affluent nations of the West. These revisionist arguments reveal one of the main problems in past approaches to poverty research; that is, they have increasingly focused on measuring poverty rather than on exploring its causal relationship to inequalities in the market place. In doing so, they obscure the debate and ask those engaged in the task to accept liberal capitalism as a given and to ignore the causes of poverty. Empirical measurement within that ideological reality thus becomes the only true epistemology of poverty and severely limits its treatment to alleviation rather than eradication.

For Canada, Sarlo (1994) argues that an *absolute* definition of poverty based on the minimum amount required to meet basic, essential human needs is the only tenable one. Unlike his early predecessors, Ames (1897) and Rowntree (1901), who were arguing for a legitimate basis for positive state intervention, Sarlo's purpose is to undermine that legitimisation. He refutes the later, *relative* definitions of poverty (for example, Marshall 1981; Runciman 1966; Townsend 1979) stating that they do not 'really measure poverty' but merely pose an argument for a greater redistribution of income from the rich to the poor. Sarlo, then, is convinced that the definition of poverty must reflect a highly visible condition characterised by severe physical and material deprivation. But this argument merely provides a convenient and entirely ideological evasion of the fundamental issue of the distribution of wealth in a democratic society.

If democracy is to mean anything beyond freedom of economic enterprise, then in its classical sense it must strive to create the conditions necessary to promote greater forms of equality (see for example, Alcock 1993; MacPherson 1965; Tawney 1961). The importance of a relative definition of poverty is that it recognises the continuum of inequality. The mere satisfaction of basic needs does not promote a healthy, democratic society in which all citizens share a basic standard of living upon which they can hope to participate meaningfully in the life of their community. The relative definition of poverty therefore, will guide the remaining analysis in this chapter.

THE INCIDENCE OF POVERTY

Because perceptions of poverty in Canada vary according to whether absolute or relative definitions are used, its measurement similarly varies. The National Council of Welfare (NCW) identified nine different measures, three of which could be said to be based on an absolute definition, the remaining six on a relative one (NCW 1996: 6–7). Statistics Canada, the federal department responsible for collecting income data in Canada, utilises a relative definition of poverty to assess income levels (Ross *et al.* 1994: 14). Beginning in 1959, it developed a measure of poverty called the low income cut-off (LICO). The LICO determines a percentage of income at which individuals and families may be said to spend a disproportionate amount on essential food, clothing and shelter, leaving little or no income for transportation, health, personal care, education, household operation, recreation or insurance. The cut-off point, however, varies by family size and the population of the city or community in which a family resides. Statistics Canada has proposed a simpler method of measuring poverty based on a purely relative definition. Under the new method there would be no adjustment based on the size of the urban or rural area. Instead, the low income cut-off would be based on 50 per cent of median gross income adjusted only for family size. It has yet to introduce this method (NCW 1996: 4; Ross *et al.* 1994: 13–15).

Using the current LICO method, in 1994 the cut-off percentage was 54.7 per cent: individuals or families who spent over that percentage of their income on essentials were considered to be poor. For example, where an individual living in a city of 500,000 or more people spent C$16,609 per year on essentials and that amount represented at least 54.7 per cent of her income she would be 'in straitened circumstances'. Or, in a city of 30,000 to 99,999 people where C$26,623 spent on essentials was 54.7 per cent or more of the income of a family of four it would be similarly categorised (Ross *et al.* 1994: 13 and 15). Although Statistics Canada does not refer to the LICO as a measure of poverty, most academics and interested organisations regard it as precisely that (Ross *et al.* 1994). The following 1994 data on poverty are therefore based on this measure and are derived from exhaustive analyses by the National Council of Welfare (1996). However, the data do not include the territories nor First Nations' populations resident on reserves within each province.

In 1994, the number of persons living in poverty in Canada was 4,795,000 or 16.6 per cent of the population. This represented a net increase of 1.3 per cent over the fifteen-year period 1980–94, but was down 0.8 per cent from 1993. During the same period, the highest incidence of poverty recorded was 18.2 per cent in 1983, the lowest, 13.6 per cent in 1989. The average incidence of poverty between 1980 and 1994 was just under 16.1 per cent (NCW 1996: 10). By province, the highest incidence of poverty in 1994 among all persons was 20.2 per cent in Québec; the lowest, 10.5 per cent in Prince Edward Island. Among the provinces with populations in excess of one million, the highest rate of poverty was in Québec, followed by Manitoba (18.4 per cent), British Columbia (16.9 per cent), Alberta (15.9 per cent) and Ontario (14.1 per cent) (NCW 1996: 20). Poverty rates were highest in cities with populations over 500,000 (families, 16.2 per cent; individuals, 42.1 per cent) and lowest in rural areas (families, 9 per cent; individuals, 22.4 per cent) (NCW 1996: 49–50).

GROUPS MOST AFFECTED BY POVERTY

By far the most disturbing poverty trends in Canada can be found among two groups: children under 18 years and single-parent mothers. The percentage of children living in poverty in Canada has risen steadily between 1980 and 1994; from 14.9 per cent (984,000) to 19.1 per cent (1,334,000). There is also a strong link between these children and the incidence of poverty among single-parent mothers under 65 years (NCW 1996: 73). Of these mothers, 57.3 per cent (317,000) were poor, a decrease of only 0.4 per cent since 1980 although down from a peak of 62.8 per cent in 1984. The greatest risk of poverty was for single-mothers with two children under 7 years: for them the rate of poverty was 82.8 per cent (NCW 1996: 17, 40–1 and 64). Of all poor single-mothers, 73 per cent relied on provincial social assistance benefits as their main source of income (NCW 1996: 64). Ironically, social assistance benefits deepen the gap and aggravate poverty in Canada. In nine provinces a single-parent with one child received less than 70 per cent of the LICO, and in three provinces less than 60 per cent (NCW 1995: 27). Finally, for two-parent families with children under 18 the poverty rate of 11.3 per cent was considerably lower than for single-mothers. However, it represented an increase of almost 2.0 per cent since 1980 (NCW 1996: 17).

Unattached persons face a higher risk of poverty in Canada than do families. For all families the general rate of poverty was 13.7 per cent (1,108,000), slightly below the general incidence of poverty in the total population. The rate of poverty for all unattached individuals in 1994, however, was 37.0 per cent (1,421,000) (NCW 1996: 14). For unattached women the rates and thus the risk were even higher: 42.6 per cent for those under 65, and 44.1 per cent for those over 65. Interestingly, the rate for women under 65 rose 4.5 per cent since 1980, while that of women 65 and over declined 24.6 per cent during the same period. Nevertheless, unattached men 65 and over face a significantly lower risk: their rate of poverty was 25.2 per cent. Similarly, the rate of poverty for unattached men under 65 years while high at 31.7 per cent was still less than that of comparable, unattached women (NCW 1996: 14 and 18).

Among Canada's retired population the rate of poverty for

persons 65 and over was 17.2 per cent (567,000), still above the
national rate. However, this represented a substantial drop from
1980, when the rate was 33.6 per cent (731,000). Improved old age
benefits have contributed to the drop in poverty among Canada's
seniors, while high unemployment, inadequate provincial social
assistance rates and low wages, especially in the services sector,
account for high poverty rates among working-age individuals and
families. Working families, for example made up 28.6 per cent of
all poor families in 1994 (NCW 1996: 13, 37–9, 69–72; Ross *et al.*
1994: 76).

Immigrants to Canada also experience a high incidence of
poverty although this has varied by year of immigration and by
family status. Immigrants who arrived in Canada between 1970 and
1979 had an average rate of poverty of 28.8 per cent. However,
among unattached persons it was 44.1 per cent while heads of
households were considerably lower at 13.6 per cent. Since 1979 the
poverty rate of immigrants has sharply increased: family heads have
a rate of 33 per cent, unattached persons, 53.4 per cent (NCW
1996: 48). One reason for this is that immigrants tend to settle in
Canada's largest cities where poverty is highest and the competition
for employment most acute (Badets 1994; Logan 1994). Because
there is usually a period of adjustment and a need to learn either
French or English, immigrants often find work first in the low-
wage service sector and thus constitute a significant proportion of
Canada's working poor (Burke 1994). A second, more ominous,
reason may lie in systemic racism and discrimination. The period of
increased unemployment among immigrants clearly coincides with
the shift from Europe to Asia, Africa and other non-Caucasian countries as sources of immigration.

Finally, a unique group who experience disproportionately high
levels of poverty are Canada's First Nations' peoples. Whether they
live on their own reserve lands or off the reserves in the cities the
great majority of them are impoverished. For example, their dependency on social assistance averaged nearly 29 per cent over the
period 1981 to 1991 or almost four times that of the general population. Moreover, the dependency rate on-reserve is over 40 per cent,
or about six times that in the general population. Finally, in 1985
the last year for which comprehensive income data were available
for First Nations, the average individual income on-reserve was
C$9,300 nearly 50 per cent less than the Canadian average and
well below the poverty lines established by the LICO. Families

on-reserve were similarly disadvantaged (Shewell and Spagnut 1995: 14, 39–40). Poverty among First Nations is a complex issue and cannot be seen wholly within the context of poverty in the mainstream market economy and the structure of the labour market. Instead, it is also related to over a century of state oppression and has as much to do with issues surrounding their own cultural and political autonomy as it does with equality and opportunity (Shewell 1991; 1995; Shewell and Spagnut 1995).

GOVERNMENT AND NON-GOVERNMENT RESPONSES TO POVERTY

Government responses

Government responses to poverty in Canada are historically slow and incremental. Relative to other western nations, Canada's performance in combating poverty has been and continues to be very weak. Particularly disturbing is Canada's inability to deal effectively with poverty among families headed by women as lone parents. Among ten industrialised nations of the west, Canada's rate of poverty for all families, for lone female parents and for young families was eighth highest, and fifth highest for two-parent families (Ross et al. 1994: 110–11 and 124).

Why is Canada's performance so weak? In part it is due to the constitutional division of powers which hinders a strong, consistent federal role in social welfare. But the Constitution and the Charter of Rights and Freedoms reflect traditional liberal values, minimising the idea of social welfare while promoting individual rights and the protection of property. In 1992, an attempt to enshrine a social charter in the Constitution ensuring the provision of social welfare programmes, full employment, and a reasonable standard of living for all Canadians was defeated in a national constitutional referendum (Canada, Supply and Services Canada 1992: 2–3). While the defeat was based on reasons associated with other proposed changes, many Canadians were obviously convinced that moving the nation closer to a social democracy was not economically sustainable or desirable.

The defeat of this amendment reaffirmed the residual framework of national social policy which, arguably, accounts mainly for Canada's inability and, indeed, its reluctance not only to alleviate but also to combat poverty at a structural level. Essentially, the state responds to poverty through income-support measures, supported by employment and incentive programmes, primarily aimed at individuals. Little is done to develop comprehensive strategies to co-ordinate the labour market with changing modes of production and emerging economic trends, strategies more common to corporatist and social democratic models of welfare state planning (Esping-Andersen 1989; Mishra 1990).

Associated with the Canadian residual response to poverty is a preoccupation with the idea of dependency. Despite the economy's volatile performance in job creation, dependency has assumed the aura of a pathology and a moral crusade: the poor and unemployed have been accused of being too reliant on the state, the result, according to right-wing thinking, of a generous, inefficient system which has induced failure, generational welfare and a culture of dependency (Battle 1994; Dean and Taylor-Gooby 1992). This reasoning serves to justify cuts in social spending as both provincial and federal governments seek ways to manage or erase deficits and debts. One method of cutting social spending has been to tighten rules of eligibility for unemployment insurance and basic welfare. Only those deemed most vulnerable and in need are to be targeted for income transfers by the state. Canada is thus returning to more selective systems of coverage and abandoning most forms of universality (Battle 1994).

One example of implicating the individual rather than combating the structural issues which produce inequality and poverty has been the implementation of work-for-welfare or *work-fare*. Under former national standards the federal government could refuse to cost-share with provinces which might attempt to introduce work as a condition for receiving basic social assistance. These standards in effect banned its occurrence (Lightman 1995). However, when the federal government began to cut back on cost-sharing and abandoned national standards under the Canada Health and Social Transfer programme, the provinces took advantage of the weakened federal presence and gradually introduced forms of workfare. At first these were voluntary (although administration pressured recipients to participate) but recently one province, Ontario, introduced compulsory work-for-welfare.

Work-for-welfare has practical, ideological and moral goals. Among them are: the development of human capital through the recipients' acquisition of work habits and skills; the enforcement of the idea of reciprocity, that is, a contract between the recipient and the government benefactor to impart the principle that there is no such thing as a 'free lunch'; and the maintenance of social order by keeping idle bodies busy and away from the lure of criminal activity (Lightman 1995: 171). As well, like prison chain gangs which allow the public to see and vicariously experience criminal punishment, so too does work-fare make a modern show of paupers both to assure and frighten the public that the state does not take dependency lightly.

Nevertheless, the extent of work-fare's effectiveness is questionable. Even those who look for empirical evidence to support the case admit to mixed results and often revert to banal moral and ideological persuasions rooted in nineteenth century assumptions about incentives and the principle of less eligibility (Krashinsky 1995; Low 1996). Since, historically, it is true in Canada that when jobs are available welfare rolls significantly decrease (Krashinsky 1995) the real issue lies in adequate levels of income coupled with training and job creation (Castonguay 1993; Low 1996; Moscovitch 1996). Governments can choose to create menial jobs, the intent of which are to shame and humiliate, or they can choose to create meaningful ones with real wages. It is not difficult to conclude therefore that the real purpose of work-fare for debt-ridden governments is its capacity to supply cheap labour for public works while simultaneously appeasing those disgruntled taxpayers who see welfare as a bottomless pit.

Non-government responses

Non-government responses to poverty mainly take the form of intellectual, policy think-tanks or populist, advocacy organisations representing both specific and broad-based interests. In most provinces there are various non-profit organisations which speak out against poverty and which work to defend and promote the interests of the poor. In addition many local charities provide services to the poor which are not provided by the state or which supplement insufficient and shrinking state programmes. Among these are shelter and support to increasing numbers of homeless persons as well as food banks for all individuals and families who are unable to nourish themselves adequately on either wages or state benefits. These provincial and municipal organisations are diverse and numerous. Their work is critical in minimising suffering and in containing the worst effects of poverty. Still, their need to exist is problematic in that poverty is depoliticised as government shirks its responsibility to combat it in meaningful ways (Riches 1997: 62–3).

At a national level several organisations are especially important in maintaining watching briefs on poverty, in providing cogent analyses of its origins and extent, and in advocating action and policies for its alleviation or elimination. Prominent among these is a quasi-government organisation, the NCW. Formed in 1969, the NCW receives its direction from a government-appointed board of private citizens, most of whom are from low income backgrounds, including welfare recipients and pensioners. The NCW acts as an advisor to the federal government on matters of concern to poor Canadians and also recommends policies which it believes would ameliorate poverty in Canada. Its most important function is the regular production of thoroughly researched publications examining a range of policies and issues which affect poverty in Canada, such as pension and tax reform, welfare benefits, universal benefits and cost-sharing. Of special importance are its annual publications on poverty profiles in Canada. Although it is a quasi-government body it is forthright in its assessment and criticism of government policies and, remarkably, has survived government down-sizing.

Other national membership organisations which provide cogent commentary, research, analysis and strong advocacy on issues of poverty in Canada include the National Action Committee on the Status of Women, the National Anti-Poverty Organisation, the Council of Canadians, the Assembly of First Nations, the Canadian Council on Social Development, and the Caledon Institute of Social Policy. These and other organisations vary considerably in their analysis of and prescribed solutions to poverty in Canada. For example, The Pan-Canadian Conference Against Poverty held in Montreal in January 1996 was attended by a range of national and provincial organisations from communist coalitions of unemployed workers to more mainstream, liberal advocacy groups. The conference naturally produced a wide discrepancy of ideas on how to end poverty from the complete overthrow of the Canadian capitalist state to the plea for just more jobs (*CPAC-Canadian Parliamentary Channel Inc.* 1996). The vastness of the country makes mobilisation of the poor difficult, so it is largely confined to local levels. However, a symbiosis often exists between national and local groups. When poor women in Québec organised a 'bread and roses' march on the provincial National Assembly, the idea took hold nationally and in June 1996 thousands of women from across the country conducted a nation-wide march culminating in Ottawa with a huge anti-poverty demonstration in front of the Parliament Buildings.

Whether this march, the anti-poverty conference, the myriad local demonstrations, the research and continuing advocacy of national and provincial organisations have any effect on Ottawa or the provinces is extremely difficult to assess. The near hegemony of private, right-wing media in Canada means that there are few publicly accessible forums where issues about poverty and its causes can be meaningfully explored and debated (Riches 1997: 75). News and information are carefully managed to minimise any outside business unease about instability and to encourage the state in its attack on welfare state measures. For example, when over 300,000 poor and working persons in Ontario demonstrated in Toronto to protest the drastic anti-labour and anti-welfare policies of the provincial government, the national daily newspaper, *The Globe and Mail*, (26 October 1996) editorially dismissed the protest. Most of the coverage towards the end of its first section downplayed the issues and simply expressed relief that there was little violence.

CONCLUSION: FUTURE PROSPECTS

The eradication of widespread poverty in Canada depends on two interrelated strategies. In the immediate short-term, the restoration and further development of state social security measures are essential. Ultimately however, in the long-term a constitutional redefinition of the state is required both to strengthen the hand of the federal government under the terms of a social charter and to enhance democratic purposes. Such a redefinition would necessarily entail a new division of powers to ensure a strong federal presence in social welfare. Both strategies, however, will be difficult to promote given the pervasiveness of right-wing ideology, the current emphasis on provincial rights (abetted by the persistent issue of Québec independence), and the absence of popular, cogent, left-wing media. Finally, the continued erosion of nation-state sovereignty as a result of the increased globalisation and mobility of capital and information further compounds the difficulty and raises alarming questions about the future responsibility for human welfare in all parts of the world (see, Guéhenno 1995).

In the short-term: an anti-poverty strategy

Battle (1994) outlines a comprehensive strategy to combat poverty which is focused on the introduction, restoration or amelioration of programmes within the existing social and economic system. Despite his concern that poverty cannot be adequately addressed without dealing with its fundamental social and economic roots, his proposals fall short of doing this. Nevertheless, his approach clearly calls for a renewed government commitment to a social safety net and that, in itself, is an important step. Battle's strategy is organised around three areas of intervention. The first area is income security. Battle rejects the idea of a guaranteed annual income and argues instead for selective, adequate and indexed income security measures for certain at risk and vulnerable populations especially the long-term unemployed, pensioners, children of low income families and, the permanently unemployable (Battle 1994: 32–4). For these groups he would seem to concede that because a smaller pie is all that's on offer it is best to make the wisest use of it possible. Consequently he proposes a realignment and re-structuring of current federal and provincial income-support programmes to meet the needs of these groups more effectively. Essentially, Battle's proposals advocate better targeting while eliminating rules which create barriers for recipients, and enforcing policies which would enhance their circumstances such as court-ordered spousal support. Finally, he recommends a more progressive tax system that would enable a better, fairer redistribution of income to the poor.

The second area of intervention, and closely tied to Battle's income-support measures, are standards and supports related to employment. Among his most important proposals are a fully-indexed, low-income tax credit, a minimum wage system constantly indexed to average wages, and the extension of employment benefits and standards to part-time employees. Historically, a glaring problem in Canada's welfare programming has been the absence of universal child-care. Probably more than any other single factor, this omission has contributed to the persistent poverty of lone mother and all low income families. Battle urges the implementation of affordable child-care but falls short of proposing a universally accessible system. His final recommendation in this area is the full implementation and enforcement of pay equity and affirmative action legislation to end any form of discrimination in both the public and private sectors of employment (Battle 1994: 34–5).

Battle's third and last area of recommended action is in education and training. Here, he proposes that employment training and upgrading be fully integrated into the educational system which must now be seen as offering life-long learning and training opportunities. Battle describes the pre-employment needs of persons on basic welfare benefits as especially important and recommends the establishment of Training and Education Access Centres across Canada to support them in entering the labour market. The government and the private employers' sector must work more closely together to identify emerging economic trends and to train the labour market to adapt to these trends. Government, he says, should accept responsibility for the education and employment preparation of those outside the labour market, while the private sector should accept a similar responsibility for those presently employed (Battle 1994: 35–6). Battle's last main proposal is to reduce unemployment through the re-invention of public works programmes or what he refers to as 'community-service jobs . . . with decent wages and benefits' which could 'produce useful goods and services . . . not available in particular communities and not supplied by the private sector' (Battle 1994: 35).

While Battle's proposals are important they are also problematic. His income-security proposals are themselves patchwork and reflect the results of a liberal society bent on particularistic, incremental planning. Most difficult are his proposals for income-testing since he implicitly surrenders any idea of universal benefits which might be supplemented by either income-tested benefits or less intrusive methods of redistribution such as a progressive income tax system. He is also quite unclear about which levels of government would assume responsibility for his proposals and indeed, precisely because they are so wide-ranging and diverse it is impossible to see how agreement would ever be reached to effect them. The main problem in the end with Battle's proposals are that they are too pragmatic and lack a clear vision of what kind of Canada Canadians might wish to live in. Battle's proposals can never transcend liberal capitalism and no matter how progressive they are in that context they thus remain vulnerable to it. The inherent ideological antagonism between liberal capitalism and social security will not disappear. In essence his proposals do not really advance democracy and fundamental principles about community, citizenship and equality. Thus, there is a need to redefine the Constitution of the Canadian state through the incorporation of a social charter.

In the long-term: a social charter

Riches (1997: 53–4) in his excellent discussion of hunger in Canada observes that the 'roots of hunger today are to be found in the structural preconditions of poverty, inequality and powerlessness, all of which are increasing'. He continues (p. 65):

If . . . hunger is . . . a political question and fundamentally a matter of economic and social rights recognised in both domestic and international law by Canada, we must ask why it is that government policy has permitted hunger to re-emerge as one of the country's significant social problems. Why is it that since the early 1980s Canadian governments of all ideological stripes turned a blind eye to the adequacy of welfare benefits, promoted punitive welfare reform proposals that exacerbated hardship, and in the mid-1990s deliberately abandoned their legislated responsibility for ensuring that the basic needs of the poorest Canadian citizens are met?

The answers are structural and ideological and have to do with how social and economic rights are understood in liberal market economies.

Riches' observation that governments of all political stripes have engaged in punitive welfare reform strikes at a telling problem in liberal democracies. They are by definition capitalist and they constitute their political systems to be so (Macpherson 1965: 4). Thus, even social democratic parties when elected to power in liberal democracies can only push the constitutional boundaries so far. Beyond a certain point the dominant business class has no tolerance for democratic freedom. The implication of this is significant. Social reform can never be truly structural only adaptive, incremental and temporary, helping the system to adjust to its own contradictions until they are corrected. What then, is to be done?

It is time for Canada to return to the idea of a social charter of rights entrenched in its constitution. When the idea was defeated in the 1992 constitutional referendum it had been lost in the debate surrounding the future of Québec in the confederation and never received the full attention it deserved. As a concept it has the potential to transform the fundamental ideological landscape of the state since it would require a redress of balance between private economic objectives and public, and social objectives. The underlying purpose of the state would no longer be primarily to protect private property and to ensure the conditions necessary for capitalism but would be broadened to ensure the health and social well-being of all Canadians based on shared national values and principles (Ontario, Ministry of Intergovernmental Affairs 1991: 14).

A social charter for Canada requires four basic elements (Ontario, Ministry of Intergovernmental Affairs 1991: 14):

- a statement of the values and principles which Canadians wish to affirm and which should guide governments in . . . social policy;
- institutions for developing, protecting, negotiating, monitoring, and enforcing policies which give concrete expression to these values and principles;
- a provision for broad public participation to ensure that policies, programmes, and services continue to be responsive to public need; and
- a recognition that national sharing is required for realising the social charter's principles across the country.

To be effective the entrenchment of a social charter in the Constitution would require a complementary amendment to the division of powers. All powers related to social welfare would have to be consolidated and shared between the federal and provincial governments, thus unconditionally legitimising the federal government's role in promoting national unity and well-being through social welfare measures.

A social charter would commit the state to social justice and greater democracy for all citizens and would minimise poverty and its worst effects. Importantly, governments could not withdraw from their social responsibilities in the name of economic imperatives. While a social charter *per se* would not change the basic economic structure of the state, it would lend the state to more collective objectives and, in the long-term, induce conditions more conducive to a social rather than a liberal democracy.

Final comments: the immediate prospects

Canada is a country with great disparities between rich and poor. Despite its abundant wealth, these will remain unless fundamental changes occur within its social, economic and political structure.

The Canadian Conference of Catholic Bishops declared in 1985 that 'the "basic contradiction of our times" rests in the "structural domination of capital . . . over people, over labour, over communities" ' (cited in Pulkingham and Ternowetsky 1996: 336). It is an assessment which remains no less true in 1996 (Pulkingham and Ternowetsky 1996: 336). Presently, the political right dominates the public agenda while the left is somewhat in disarray. Indeed, it has been fighting a rearguard action since the collapse of the Soviet Union armed the ideological right to ridicule policies that it could associate with socialism. Thus, the current prospects for combating poverty in Canada on the scale that is required are not hopeful (Battle 1994: 37; Riches 1997). However, even if the goals of the short-term are to be achieved, then according to Pulkingham and Ternowetsky (1996) the first task is to influence public opinion again so that poverty, social policy and social programmes become the focus of the public agenda and the centre of full and fair debate.

REFERENCES

Alcock, P. (1993) *Understanding Poverty*, London: Macmillan.

Ames, H.B. (1897, 1972) *The City Below the Hill*, Toronto: University of Toronto Press.

Badets, J. (1994) 'Canada's Immigrants: Recent Trends', in *Canadian Social Trends: A Canadian Studies Reader* (Vol. 2), Toronto: Thompson Educational Publishing.

Banting, K.G. (1987) *The Welfare State and Canadian Federalism* (2nd edn), Kingston and Montreal: McGill-Queen's University Press.

Barlow, M. (1996) 'Seven Years of Free Trade', *Canadian Perspectives* (Spring): 7.

Barlow, M. and Campbell, B. (1995) *Straight Through the Heart: How the Liberals Abandoned the Just Society*, Toronto: Harper Collins.

Battle, K. (1994) 'Poverty and the Welfare State', in Samuelson, L. (ed.) *Power and Resistance: Critical Thinking About Canadian Social Issues*, Halifax: Fernwood Publishing.

Biggs, B. and Bollman, R. (1994) 'Urbanization in Canada', in *Canadian Social Trends: A Canadian Studies Reader* (vol. 2), Toronto: Thompson Educational Publishing.

Burke, M.A. (1994) 'Canada's Immigrant Children', in *Canadian Social Trends: A Canadian Studies Reader* (vol. 2), Toronto: Thompson Educational Publishing.

Canada, Statistics Canada (1996) *Population Data for Census Metropolitan Areas, July 1995*, Ottawa: Statistics Canada.

Canada, Supply and Services Canada (1992) *Consensus Report on the Constitution*, Ottawa: Supply and Services Canada.

Canadian Conference of Catholic Bishops (1985) 'Moral Vision and Political Will', in Drache, D. and Cameron, C. (eds) *The Other Macdonald Report*, Toronto: James Lorimer.

Castonguay, C. (1993), 'Income Support and Social Dependency', in Reynolds, E.B. (ed.) *Income Security in Canada: Changing Needs, Changing Means*, Montreal: The Institute for Research on Public Policy.

Cook, R. (1985) *The Regenerators: Social Criticism in Late Victorian English Canada*, Toronto: University of Toronto Press.

Copp, T. (1974) *The Anatomy of Poverty: The Condition of the Working Class in Montreal, 1897–1929*, Toronto: McClelland and Stewart.

CPAC-Canadian Parliamentary Channel Inc. (1996) 'The Pan-Canadian Conference Against Poverty', Montreal (January) *Televised Proceedings*.

Dean, H. and Taylor-Gooby, P. (1992) *Dependency Culture: The Explosion of a Myth*, Hempstead: Harvester Wheatsheaf.

Esping-Andersen, G. (1989) 'The Three Political Economies of the Welfare State', *The Canadian Review of Sociology and Anthropology* 26 (1): 10–36.

Finkel, A. (1977) 'Origins of the welfare state in Canada', in Panitch, L. (ed.) *The Canadian State: Political Economy and Political Power*, Toronto: University of Toronto Press.

Geller, G. and Joel, J. (1996) 'Struggling For Citizenship in The Global Economy: Bond Raters Versus Women And Children', in Pulkingham J. and Ternowetsky, G. (eds) *Remaking Canadian Social Policy: Social Security in the Late 1990s*, Halifax: Fernwood Publishing.

Guéhenno, J. (1995) *The End of the Nation-State*, Minneapolis: University of Minnesota Press.

Guest, D. (1985) *The Emergence of Social Security in Canada* (rev. edn), Vancouver: University of British Columbia Press.

Haddow, R.S. (1993) *Poverty Reform in Canada 1958–1978: State and Class Influences on Policy Making*, Kingston and Montreal: McGill-Queen's University Press.

Hobsbawm, E.J. (1990) *Nations and Nationalism Since 1780: Programme, Myth, Reality*, Cambridge: Cambridge University Press.

Irving, A. (1987) 'Federal-Provincial Issues in Social Policy', in Yelaja, S. (ed.) *Canadian Social Policy* (rev. edn), Waterloo: Wilfrid Laurier University Press.

Krashinsky, M. (1995) 'Putting the Poor to Work: Why 'Workfare' is an Idea whose Time has Come', in Richards, J. and Watson, W.G. (eds) *Helping the Poor: A Qualified Case for 'Workfare'* (The Social Policy Challenge Series 5), Toronto: C.D. Howe Institute.

Laxer, G. (1995) 'Social Solidarity, Democracy and Global Capitalism', *Canadian Review of Sociology and Anthropology* 32 (3): 287–313.

Lightman, E. S. (1995) 'You Can Lead a Horse to Water; but . . . : The Case Against Workfare in Canada', in Richards, J. and Watson, W.G. (eds), *Helping the Poor: A Qualified Case for 'Workfare'* (The Social Policy Challenge Series 5), Toronto: C.D. Howe Institute.

Logan, R. (1994) 'Immigration During the 1980's', in *Canadian Social Trends: A Canadian Studies Reader* (vol. 2), Toronto: Thompson Educational Publishing.

Low, W. (1996) 'Wide of the Mark: Using 'Targeting' and Work Incentives to Direct Social Assistance to Single Parents', in Pulkingham J. and Ternowetsky, G. (eds), *Remaking Canadian Social Policy: Social Security in the Late 1990s*, Halifax: Fernwood Publishing.

MacPherson, C.B. (1965) *The Real World of Democracy* (The Massey Lectures, Fourth Series), Toronto: C.B.C. Enterprises.

—— (1977) *The Life and Times of Liberal Democracy*, Oxford: Oxford University Press.

Marshall, T.H. (1981) 'Changing Ideas about Poverty', in *The Right to Welfare and Other Essays*, New York: The Free Press.

McKie, C. (1994) 'Population Ageing: Baby Boomers into the 21st Century', in *Canadian Social Trends: A Canadian Studies Reader* (vol. 2), Toronto: Thompson Educational Publishing.

McNaught, K. (1988) *The Penguin History of Canada* (rev. edn), London: Penguin Books.

Mishra, R. (1990) *The Welfare State in Capitalist Society: Policies of Retrenchment and Maintenance in Europe, North America and Australia*, Toronto: University of Toronto Press.

Morton, D. (1983) *A Short History of Canada*, Edmonton: Hurtig.

Moscovitch, A. (1996) 'Canada Health and Social Transfer: What was Lost?', *Canadian Review of Social Policy* 37 (Spring): 66–75.

Moscovitch, A. and Drover, G. (1987) 'Social Expenditures and the Welfare State: The Canadian Experience in Historical Perspective', in Moscovitch, A. and Albert, J. (eds) *The 'Benevolent' State: The Growth of Welfare in Canada*, Toronto: Garamond Press.

Myles, J. (1988) 'Decline or Impasse? The Current State of the Welfare State', *Studies in Political Economy* 26 (Summer): 73–107.

National Council of Welfare (NCW) (1995) *Welfare Incomes 1994*, Ottawa: Supply and Services Canada.

—— (1996) *Poverty Profile 1994*, Ottawa: Supply and Services Canada.

Naylor, R.T. (1987) *Canada in the European Age 1453–1919*, Vancouver: New Star Books.

O'Neill, J. (1994) 'Changing Occupational Structure', in *Canadian Social Trends: A Canadian Studies Reader* (vol. 2), Toronto: Thompson Educational Publishing.

Ontario, Ministry of Intergovernmental Affairs (1991) *A Canadian Social Charter: Making Our Shared Values Stronger* (Discussion Paper), Toronto: Ministry of Intergovernmental Affairs.

Owram, D. (1986) *The Government Generation: Canadian Intellectuals and the State 1900–1945*, Toronto: University of Toronto Press.

Parliament, J. (1994) 'Labour Force Trends: Two Decades in Review', in *Canadian Social Trends: A Canadian Studies Reader* (vol. 2), Toronto: Thompson Educational Publishing.

Prentice, A., Bourne, P., Cuthbert-Brandt, G., Light, B., Mitchinson, W. and Black, N. (1988), *Canadian Women: A History*, Toronto: Harcourt Brace Jovanovich.

Pulkingham J. and Ternowetsky, G. (1996) 'Social Policy Choices and the Agenda for Change', in Pulkingham, J. and Ternowetsky, G. (eds)

Remaking Canadian Social Policy: Social Security in the Late 1990s, Halifax: Fernwood Publishing.

Riches, G. (1997) 'Hunger in Canada: Abandoning the Right to Food', in Riches, G. (ed.) *First World Hunger: Food Security and Welfare Politics*, London: Macmillan.

Ross, D.P., Shillington, E.R. and Lochhead, C. (1994) *The Canadian Fact Book on Poverty – 1994*, Ottawa: The Canadian Council on Social Development.

Rowntree, B.S. (1901), *Poverty: A Study of Town Life*, London: Macmillan.

Runciman, W.G. (1966) *Relative Deprivation and Social Justice*, London: Routledge and Kegan Paul.

Sarlo, C.A. (1994), 'Poverty in Canada – 1994', *Fraser Forum: Critical Issues Bulletin*, Vancouver: The Fraser Institute.

Schellenberg, G. (1996) 'Diversity In Retirement And The Financial Security Of Older Workers', in Pulkingham, J. and Ternowetsky, G. (eds) *Remaking Canadian Social Policy: Social Security in the Late 1990s*, Halifax: Fernwood Publishing.

Scott, K. (1996) 'The Dilemma of Liberal Citizenship: Women and Social Assistance Reform in the 1990s', *Studies in Political Economy* 50 (Summer): 7–36.

Shewell, H. (1991) 'The Use of Social Assistance for Employment Creation on Indian Reserves: An Appraisal', in Cassidy, F. and Seward, S. B. (eds) *Alternatives to Social Assistance in Indian Communities*, Halifax: The Institute for Research on Public Policy.

—— (1995), *Origins of Contemporary Indian Social Welfare in the Canadian Liberal State: An Historical Case Study in Social Policy, 1873–1965* (PhD dissertation), Toronto: University of Toronto.

Shewell, H. and Spagnut, A. (1995) 'The First Nations of Canada: Social Welfare and the Quest for Self-government', in Dixon, J. and Scheurell, R.P. (eds) *Social Welfare With Indigenous Peoples*, London: Routledge.

Shields, J. and McBride, S. (1994) 'Dismantling a Nation: The Canadian Political Economy and Continental Free Trade', in Samuelson, L. (ed.) *Power and Resistance: Critical Thinking About Canadian Social Issues*, Halifax: Fernwood Publishing.

Silver, S. (1996) 'The Struggle for National Standards: Lessons from the Federal Role in Health Care', in Pulkingham, J. and Ternowetsky, G. (eds) *Remaking Canadian Social Policy: Social Security in the Late 1990s*, Halifax: Fernwood Publishing.

Simeon, R. and Robinson, I. (1990) *State, Society, and the Development of Canadian Federalism* (The Collected Research Studies for the Royal Commission on the Economic Union and Development Prospects for Canada. Volume 71), Toronto: University of Toronto Press.

Struthers, J. (1983) *No Fault of Their Own: Unemployment and the Canadian Welfare State 1914–1941*, Toronto: University of Toronto Press.

Tawney, R.H. (1961) *Equality* (rev. 4th edn), New York: Capricorn Books.

Teeple, G. (1995) *Globalization and the Decline of Social Reform*, Toronto: Garamond Press.

Ternowetsky, G. and Riches, G. (1993) *Labour Market Restructuring and the Public Safety Net: Current Trends in the Australian and Canadian Welfare*

State (Working Paper No. 9), University of Regina, Social Administration Research Unit.

Townsend, P. (1979) *Poverty in the United Kingdom: A Survey of Household Resources and Standards of Living*, London: Allen Lane.

Watkins, M. (1992) *Madness and Ruin: Politics and the Economy in the Neoconservative Age*, Toronto: Between The Lines.

Chapter 4

Hong Kong

Stewart MacPherson

The six million people of tiny Hong Kong have the fourth highest gross domestic product (GDP) per capita in the world (HK$189,400 or some US$25,000), after the US, Switzerland and Kuwait. In the March 1997 budget the government announced a projected surplus of HK$31.7 billion for 1997–8 and accumulated reserves of HK$359 billion by March 1998. But despite Hong Kong's economic achievements over the past three decades, poverty remains an important issue. Hong Kong has been transformed from a city of poor migrants in the 1960s into one of the most affluent and influential cities of the world in the 1990s. The growth of prosperity has been extraordinary and made possible by the conjunction of many factors. Initially, cheap labour for manufacturing in Hong Kong itself, and more recently from the employment by many Hong Kong companies of cheap labour in southern China.

But many people in Hong Kong are poor; some 575,000 by one estimate (MacPherson and Lo 1997) or 640,000 people by another estimate (Wong and Chua 1996) – about 11 per cent of the population. A group which particularly experiences severe difficulties and underlines many features of Hong Kong's economic success and transition are new immigrants from China. Typically these are the wives and children of low-paid workers. Wives and children of Hong Kong citizens may enter from the mainland at the discretion of the Hong Kong government. But wives and children of mainland men living in Hong Kong are subject to two major restrictions. First they must apply to the authorities in China for one-way entry permits before they can go to live in Hong Kong. Second, there is a quota of 150 one-way permit holders per day allowed to enter Hong Kong; 54,000 a year.

Getting these permits in China is difficult, and often expensive.

Corruption and bribery are widespread and in many cases mothers and children are not allowed to emigrate to Hong Kong at the same time, with children often gaining approval first. When young children are approved to enter without their mothers, fathers may have to give up their jobs to care for them, causing severe financial strain. Inevitably the situation puts significant emotional and psychological pressure on the families. New immigrant families are among the poorest in the community, not least because most remain ineligible for public housing, under the rule that half of all family members must have been resident in Hong Kong for seven years to qualify. Only people over the age of 60 may qualify for 'compassionate re-housing' outside this rule. Forced into the private rented sector, they can often afford only the most overcrowded and squalid accommodation, but even that at a very high cost.

It is not known for sure what effect the change of Hong Kong's status to a Special Administrative Region (SAR) of China will have on the rate of inward migration of wives and children. Potentially, the numbers are huge. Latest Hong Kong government estimates are of 400,000 wives and children taking up their newly acquired right of residence after 1 July 1997. As most of the men in these families are in low-paid employment the implications are severe. Beyond the 400,000 who will automatically have rights of residence, there are potentially many hundreds of thousands more who could seek entry to Hong Kong. It is certain that China will continue to control the granting of one-way entry permits. What is less certain is whether the Hong Kong SAR government will retain autonomous control of the entry quota. If present controls of internal migration into special economic zones within China can be taken as a guide, all control of policy in this regard will be with Beijing.

The migration of poor workers and their families is a major issue for all cities in poor countries. Hong Kong has for many years avoided the massive problems faced by other cities, essentially because of the maintenance of the border with China. To what extent this will continue to be so is one of the most significant questions over the future of poverty and social assistance.

Hong Kong's affluence points up the severity of its poverty. The housing of the poorest is appalling – in public housing the minimum standard is restricted to less than 5 square metres per head, and in the private sector it can be very much less. The conditions, especially in the private sector are generally squalid. Possessions are very few and social activity is minimal. For the elderly, who are the great majority of the poorest, life is very hard indeed. Many work, at anything which can raise even the most meagre amount, for as long as they are physically able. As Hong Kong has become more affluent, all the questions of 'relative' poverty have been raised. But, important as these are, there is much absolute poverty yet to be dealt with adequately.

The discussion in this chapter examines the issue from two perspectives. The first is in terms of the nature and extent of poverty in Hong Kong. The second is in relation to the government's social assistance scheme – Comprehensive Social Security Assistance (CSSA).

THE BACKGROUND TO POVERTY IN HONG KONG

Hong Kong is quintessentially a city of migrants. About half of the six million permanent residents of Hong Kong were born in China and most migrated to Hong Kong in the late 1950s and 1960s. Some controlled migration has continued ever since. Except for those fleeing the communist victory in China, the great majority of migrants were from poor, and usually rural backgrounds in China. They came to Hong Kong with virtually nothing except their dreams of a new life and their determination to succeed. They lived in appalling conditions. From the 1950s through the 1970s they lived in slums and squatter settlements as found in Manila and Bangkok. They, and successive migrants, eventually moved into extremely basic public housing, with shared toilets and shared kitchens, and very little space per person, as this accommodation became available from the 1960s onwards. As Hong Kong became more affluent standards rose, and the children of poor migrants were able to get education and employment. Many poor migrants themselves achieved economic success, either in Hong Kong itself or overseas, as many hundreds of thousands moved onward to the US, Canada, Australia and elsewhere. As the economy grew so did wages and consumption. In the mid-1990s the GDP per capita began to outstrip the countries of Europe, by 1997 it had exceeded that of the UK, the colonial power. Patterns of expenditure and consumption in the 1990s are, for a large part of the population, modelled on the US and Japan. The shopping mall is an integral part of the new private ownership housing developments. Housing itself has come to symbolise the scale of personal incomes. Even relatively modest apartments are bought by couples in middle range employment for prices around £375,00 to £500,000 (HK$4.7 million to HK$6.3 million). The culture of Hong Kong is dominated by materialism, individualism and consumerism.

This history – of a massive shift from a colony of migrant peasants in squatter settlements to a world city of affluent consumers, feted by the world for their success – is of tremendous importance in understanding poverty in Hong Kong. Faith in an unfettered market is profound, as is the belief in unlimited opportunities for the individual. But more than that there is the contrast with the past as a constant theme, a reminder constantly made, that very many very poor migrants made a success of the opportunities of Hong Kong. The message is therefore that those who are without resources now can surely do the same. However unrealistic this may be it a very powerful force indeed. As with views on the nature of the society then so too with opinions on the poverty level itself. Many of the most influential carry with them the concepts of the past, and not least the notions of poverty relevant to the slums and settlements of the earlier era. In these terms poverty means starvation, disease, extreme squalor and the hopelessness and despair of abject poverty. However irrelevant these concepts may be in a community with GDP per capita at a higher level than the UK, they are a powerful reality. They are buttressed, and will be increasingly so in the future, by definitions of poverty in the People's Republic of China. China is a poor, predominantly rural society, engaged in a massive and traumatic shift to an urbanised, industrialised market driven economy. But now, and for a long time to come, the levels of consumption across China will remain closer to those of Third World countries than to Hong Kong. Definitions of poverty in China are rooted in the realities of the Chinese economy and society. They vary from country to town and from city to city, but even in the most affluent cities of southern China poverty concepts and definitions remain firmly rooted to restricted subsistence. The social assistance programmes which are associated with these poverty concepts are reminiscent of the Poor Law at the time of industrial transformation in Europe 200 years ago.

The influence of China must not be underestimated. It is very powerful, in many areas of life in Hong Kong, and most definitely in social policy. There are two major forms that this influence takes, both having great effect – the real and the imagined. Real influence is already apparent in the policy statements of the Beijing appointed Chief executive designate, Tung Chee-hwa, who has already made it very clear that although Hong Kong will have a degree of autonomy under the 'one country two systems' principle, that autonomy will be circumscribed by the need to avoid offence to Beijing. Real influence is also clear in statements from Beijing on social issues. In March 1997 two statements were made which may indicate the direction of mainland influence. The first was that in future there would be unrestricted entry from the mainland to Hong Kong. This potentially devastating change of policy was tempered by the assurance that exit from the mainland would continue to be strictly controlled, but it nonetheless marks a dramatic shift. The second example declares a willingness to interfere in the affairs of the future Special Administrative Region which goes well beyond past assurances. The Chinese Foreign Ministry declared that a number of books in use in Hong Kong schools would need to be revised after July 1997 as they were ideologically unsound. It is not the content of the books which is the issue, they may well be inaccurate and in need of change, but the willingness of Beijing to interfere.

These examples are important in themselves, but from the point of view of the present topic they are important in underlining the strength of Beijing's influence in general. This is relevant to the second major form of influence – the imagined, which may in fact be much more powerful. In many spheres, it has become clear that people in Hong Kong are making assumptions about what Beijing thinks and may do, and basing their decisions upon these assumptions. This is a complex and subtle game, with far reaching consequences. In social policy it means second guessing of a high order. In relation to poverty and the public support of the poor, it means taking the few, rather hostile, statements on the topics that have actually been made from Beijing and weaving them with many strands of assumption, hearsay and guesswork to produce a cloth of great strength if not of beauty. Thus, what is 'acceptable' to China becomes a touchstone of poverty and social assistance discussions. But at levels other than explicit policy discussion, in terms of people's perceptions of poverty and welfare, the China factor clearly has a powerful effect. It may only be legitimating views already held, but it is a powerful influence nonetheless.

Perceptions of poverty in Hong Kong are complex. They are profoundly shaped by the post war history of the territory, not least by the transformation of poor migrants to world class consumers. They are greatly influenced by China. These perceptions of poverty can be seen in the debate on the definition and measurement of poverty that have taken place in Hong Kong in recent years.

POVERTY AND SOCIAL ASSISTANCE

While Hong Kong has achieved great wealth and continuing high rates of economic growth, the rights of the poorest are neglected. The common perception is that Hong Kong people enjoy uniquely open opportunities for upward social mobility, which means that the problems of poverty are generally underestimated or unrecognised, certainly by the better off groups. The conventional wisdom is that these views of poverty are shared throughout the society.

In recent years, the gap between the rich and the poor has grown wider, while the size of the poor population has increased rapidly. In 1971, the poorest 20 per cent of households shared 6.2 per cent of all household income, while the richest 20 per cent shared 49.3 per cent. But by 1991, the poorest 20 per cent had only 4.3 per cent, while the richest 20 per cent's share had increased to 52.8 per cent (Ngan 1996).

The number of people receiving social assistance has increased dramatically in recent years, to about 160,000 households (about 200,000 people) at the beginning of 1997. The number is expected to rise to at least 180,00 by mid-1997. This would be almost 10 per cent of Hong Kong's two million households. One cause of this increase is the relocation of many Hong Kong manufacturing industries to southern China, with the number of workers in such factories in Hong Kong declining from close to one million in 1981 to under 400,000 in 1995. As a consequence, women, middle-aged and elderly workers have suffered from decreases in real wages, under-employment and difficulties in finding new employment.

The elderly population is especially vulnerable to poverty and the number of people aged over 60 is projected to grow from 7.4 to 18.1 per cent of the total population by 2011. The inadequacy of the pension system is an important factor, and very many older people rely on social assistance payments.

Social assistance in Hong Kong is facing potential crisis as the number of recipients grows, and debates on the levels of allowance force rates to higher (though still grossly inadequate) levels. In the five years to 1996–7, expenditure on social assistance has risen from HK$1 billion to HK$6 billion. Shifting attitudes will make the poor more willing to apply for relief, thus adding further to the demand for assistance. Over all of this, the long-term future of assistance is inevitably affected by the transition to Special Administrative Region status in mid-1997.

Background to social assistance in Hong Kong

In 1948 the Hong Kong colonial government was forced, by the desperate circumstances of many migrants, to offer public assistance for the first time. The extreme levels of poverty and destitution were such as to make continued inaction impossible. The introduction of extremely restricted public assistance, in kind rather than cash, and with considerable exclusions, was common in the colonies (MacPherson 1982). The official colonial position was made clear in a 1965 policy paper and, as is so often the case, it was a convenient conjunction of cultural sensitivity and cost-saving. The policy was to 'maintain Chinese traditions', which treated poverty, infirmity and natural disaster as personal matters to be dealt with by the family system. But pressure to do something about the obvious problems of poverty was mounting. In 1966, the British government sent Lady Gertrude Williams, to advise. Her advice was that the capacity of the extended family system was no longer capable of carrying out its traditional functions of caring for the old, the young, the disabled and the unemployed as it had in the past. There was, she argued, a need for social insurance, even if on a limited basis (Jones 1990: 173). In the short-term, a social insurance scheme could cover risks to the breadwinner from illness and death; in the longer run, the difficulties faced in older age. The Hong Kong government responded by appointing a working party. It reported that there should be progressive development of social security, based on social insurance. The insurance system was to be complemented by 'a modern and uniform system of public assistance from public funds' (Hong Kong Government 1967).

The recommendations were not followed. Instead, in 1971, the Hong Kong government introduced a means-tested public assistance scheme that would deliver benefits in cash. This was the first time the state had done so in Hong Kong. It took over responsibility for cash assistance from voluntary agencies. The scheme was set up in such a way as to minimise cost, and was modelled on the UK National Assistance (Heppell 1974; Heppell and Webb 1973). Hong Kong moved into the 1970s, a period of unprecedented economic growth and rapid modernisation, with no pension or provident fund programmes and an embryonic social security system based on the Poor Law.

Comprehensive social security assistance

In Hong Kong, social assistance remains the only state social security payment of subsistence income (see Table 4.1). It has not changed in its essentials since its introduction in 1971. In principle, all those in financial need are eligible, including those in employment at low earnings, but recipients of assistance (since 1993 renamed Comprehensive Social Security Assistance – CSSA) are mainly older people. The basic rates are intended to cover all essential requirements.

Besides the basic rates, supplementary allowances may be paid, such as old age supplement and disability supplement. There is a long-term supplement paid to those who have received assistance

Table 4.1 Social security in Hong Kong

Programmes	Eligible recipients
CSSA Scheme	Means-tested. Any person whose income and resources are below the prescribed level
Social Security Allowance Scheme	
Normal Old Age Allowance	Any person 65–9
Higher Old Age Allowance	Any person aged 70 or more
Normal Disability Allowance	Any severely disabled person
Higher Disability Allowance	Any severely disabled person requiring constant attendance
Accident Compensation Schemes	Any work accident victim
Emergency Relief	Any victim of natural and other disasters
Criminal and Law Enforcement Injuries Compensation Scheme	Any person injured, disabled or killed due to a crime of violence or law enforcement
Traffic Accident Victims Assistance Scheme	Any victim of a traffic accident

for more than 12 months. Special grants cover the cost of accommodation and certain special expenses (for example extra dietary
requirements). In 1995–6 the total expenditure was just over
HK$4,236 million, an increase of just under 25 per cent over the
previous year. It is estimated that it will exceed HK$6 million in
1996–7. There were 170,000 cases in March 1997, up from
102,000 in 1994 (about 200,000 people were dependent on public
assistance in early 1997).

Since the early 1990s there has been a dramatic shift in the
pattern of social security expenditure. As Table 4.2 shows total
expenditure on CSSA in absolute terms and as a percentage of total
social welfare expenditure have risen dramatically.

Moreover, there are more than twice as many cases in 1996 as
there were five years ago (see Table 4.3).

If judged by the wealth and income levels of the community, the
rates of payment are low. The basic rate from April 1996 was
HK$1,615 per month up to age 59, and HK$1,935 for those 60–9,
with higher rates for those over 70 and those with disabilities.

In 1997, the attitudes to the relief of poverty and to income
maintenance are reflected in government policy are as they were 25
years ago. Protection from hardship and poverty relies on self-help
and on the family. The role of government social security is to meet

Table 4.2 Expenditure on social assistance: 1991–2 to 1995–6

Year	Expenditure on PA/CSSA (HK$m)	PA/CSSA expenditure as percentage of total social welfare expenditure
1990–1	960	16.5
1991–2	1,136	16.4
1992–3	1,409	18.0
1993–4	2,443	26.6
1994–5	3,427	31.3
1995–6	4,236	29.0

Source: Hong Kong Social Welfare Department.

Table 4.3 Social assistance cases: 1971–96

Year (as at September)	PA/CSSA cases	Cases as percentage of total population
1971	11,240	0.3
1974	35,610	0.8
1977	47,671	1.3
1980	45,274	0.9
1983	53,785	1.0
1986	62,172	1.1
1989	65,252	1.1
1990	67,733	1.2
1991	69,640	1.2
1992	77,211	1.3
1993	88,634	1.5
1994	102,455	1.7
1995	122,062	2.0
1996 (March)	136,201	2.2

Source: Hong Kong Social Welfare Department.

only the most basic needs of the most deserving, in the direst need of financial assistance. Public assistance has been seen as a safety net for those unable to support themselves and without relatives willing to support them. In Hong Kong it is a policy of absolute minimum expenditure, and minimum intervention in the market or the systems of family obligation.

Poverty, social assistance and social change

The number of people dependent on social assistance continues to grow. The greatest rates of growth is in the unemployed and those with low incomes (up 55 per cent and 74 per cent respectively in the year to January 1997), but the elderly remain by far the biggest single group, and their numbers are still increasing steadily (see Table 4.4).

In Hong Kong, as in many other societies, government refuses to adopt an official poverty line despite being pressured to do so. In an answer to a question in the Legislative Council in early 1995, the Secretary for Health and Welfare said: 'There appears to be a general consensus amongst experts that "poverty" as such defies definition – whether in absolute or relative terms or by any other more subjective method'.

In such circumstances the prevailing level of support through social assistance is commonly taken as a *de facto* or official poverty line, if government claims, as it does in Hong Kong, that rates of social assistance are adequate, and those receiving social assistance are therefore not in poverty. This puts attention on the specific rates of social assistance support. When the level of social assistance payments is considered, a fundamental question is – how much is enough? In Hong Kong, social assistance dominates social security. Nearly all governments intend non-contributory, means-tested social assistance to be a last resort benefit targeted at the poorest

Table 4.4 CSSA cases by type: 1993–4 to 1995–6

Category	1993–4	1994–5	1995–6
Elderly	61,026	72,468	84,243
Blind	946	444	460
Deaf	338	93	143
Physically disabled	2,644	1,982	2,543
Mentally ill	5,687	5,832	6,912
Temporary illness	10,072	11,308	14,450
Single-parent family	6,134	6,453	8,982
Low earnings	1,407	991	1,814
Unemployed	3,876	5,302	10,131
Others	2,974	4,588	6,523
Total	95,104	109,461	136,201
(New applications)	(36,066)	(49,906)	(63,154)

Source: Hong Kong Social Welfare Department.

and most disadvantaged members of the community, those with the least access to alternative sources of support. A key question for policy-makers is to determine the level of social assistance payments. Social assistance for those without alternative resources must be at a rate that is considered adequate to meet standard individual and family requirements. So the key question becomes 'how much is enough?'

The level of social assistance and estimates of the number in poverty

In November 1996, a visiting United Nations group monitoring compliance with the International Covenant on Economic, Social and Cultural Rights pressed the Hong Kong government to increase spending on social security. One of the issues the group raised was the low level of social assistance payments, relative to the level of financial reserves. Such criticism is not new, and has been increasing in recent years.

In the early 1990s there was much criticism of the social assistance scheme from academics, social welfare agencies, community groups, and legislative councillors themselves. In 1993 the Legislative Council Welfare Services Panel called for a review of the adequacy of the public assistance rates (Ngan 1993). The task passed to the Hong Kong Council of Social Service, the co-ordinating body of welfare agencies in Hong Kong. The Council in turn invited an academic to undertake the review. The work was undertaken between mid-1993 and mid-1994 as a piece of independent research (MacPherson 1994; Sequiera *et al.* 1996).

To establish current CSSA standards of living, there was a survey of a stratified random sample of 683 households receiving CSSA in March 1994. Overall, the survey shows that even though they are spending 70 per cent of their income on food, households dependent on CSSA are spending less than is needed on food. To achieve this level of food expenditure, they are drastically reducing expenditure on all other items.

The consequences, especially for families with children, are extreme restrictions on social activity and participation in the normal activities of ordinary people in Hong Kong. Household possessions are meagre, diets are minimal, clothing and footwear are at extremely low levels. The rates of CSSA were clearly inadequate for the maintenance of a decent minimum standard of living. Total monthly expenditure in 70 per cent of the households surveyed was in the range HK$500–HK$1,400 per month per person. Overall average total expenditure was just over HK$1,100 per month per person.

Expenditure on food is always the largest single item in all low income budgets. In the case of CSSA households, studies have shown that food takes between 60 and 70 per cent of expenditure. The average amount spent per person on food prepared at home each month was around HK$600. To this must be added an amount for food eaten outside the home. For the majority, without subsidised food, the mean level of monthly expenditure on food per person was HK$730, with three-quarters spending less than $920 per month per person. Comparing the figures for food expenditure with those for total expenditure CSSA recipients are spending around 70 per cent of their total expenditure on food. This is a very high proportion; less than 30 per cent is usual for poor households in developed societies.

The research concluded that the rates of social assistance were far too low, especially for children and single-parents. Inadequate rates contribute to considerable hardship, and in particular to very severe restrictions on social activity. For children, these conditions had serious consequences. Poverty in Hong Kong is not a matter of individual failure or family dysfunction. It is, rather, a consequence of the effects of socio-economic change on particularly vulnerable groups. Lui and Wong, the authors of a wide ranging research study in the mid-1990s concluded (1995: 35): 'vulnerable households face many problems. Once they are unemployed, displaced or get sick, the other problems will come one after another.'

The work generated new recommended rates. In June 1994 the results of the research, and the recommended rates, were published. In the ensuing debate, groups representing and supporting CSSA recipients argued strenuously with government representatives over the adequacy of the CSSA rates. The Legislative Council's Welfare Services Panel then urged government to adopt new CSSA rates as recommended in the research report. The Health and Welfare Branch, responsible for social security considered the report and its findings in very great detail. In September 1994 they rejected the findings, because they thought a budget standards approach was inappropriate and that the financial implications of raising the rates to the recommended levels would be damaging to the Hong Kong economy. Pressure continued on the government to do something about the rates. In October 1994 Hong Kong's last Governor, Christopher Patten, announced in his policy speech that there would be small increases for children and single-parents, from April 1995. A government review was announced, which was expected to report at the end of 1995. In the event Patten anticipated the review in his 1995 policy address. The review had found that the CSSA rates were not adequate and improvements were to take effect from April 1996. The most significant of these were increases of around 60 per cent in the standard monthly rates for single-parents and those claimants in ill-health. The increase for the unemployed was only 33 per cent, because rates had to kept at levels that would not provide a disincentive to work.

The Report on the Review of the Comprehensive Social Security Assistance (CSSA) scheme was released in March 1996 (Hong Kong Government 1996). Many aspects of the scheme were reviewed besides the basic rates. A number of changes were proposed in the administration of the scheme and in the detail of specific allowances. The basic philosophy of the scheme and the general approach to allowances however remained the same. After the review a detailed assessment of the CSSA scheme, carried out by the research section of the Legislative Council (Liu *et al*. 1996: executive summary, para. 7) concluded that: '[t]he total assistance received by CSSA recipients is *not* sufficient to cover the monthly expenses under the conditions of Hong Kong'.

The financial implications of the reforms proposed in the Review were just over HK$508 million, of which HK$317 was attributable to changes in the standard rates. So, relatively little was done for the poorest in Hong Kong and overall the rates remained at levels that were adequate for subsistence but little else. Thus the *de facto* poverty line remains very low and essentially informed by a restricted concept of 'basic needs'. The essence of the Hong Kong government approach remained intact. Although the review identified many important issues, it dealt with relatively few.

At the end of 1996 a new analysis of the official 1994–5 Household Expenditure data was undertaken and published by the Hong Kong Council of Social Services (Wong and Chua 1996). This was the data that was previously used by the government to support its refusal to raise the rates of social assistance beyond what was claimed to be an adequate level for basic needs. What the government had done was to compare the expenditure patterns of CSSA recipients with the lowest 5 per cent group in the income distribution who were not receiving social assistance. There had been criticism of this approach, but the government countered by asserting that its findings that CSSA recipients spent more on food was true, as much as that of the 20 per cent group in the income distribution. Wong and Chua (1996) used a different approach to the same data and found that households in the lowest income groups – 0–5 per cent, 5–10 per cent and 10–15 per cent – spent more on food as their incomes rose, until a point was reached when the proportion of food spending began to drop. They argue that the presence of such a 'turning point' suggests that spending on food is suppressed at very low income levels. Thus, they argued that these households are in 'abject poverty' as they are unable to meet basic and necessary food expenditure from their incomes. Wong and Chua argue that the government's 'basic needs' approach in determining the level of CSSA payments, and incidentally setting the *de facto* poverty line, is essentially an exercise in the subjective judgements of officials. The 'poverty threshold' approach, they claim is more realistic because it more closely reflects households' actual needs and expenditures. Using this approach, Wong and Chua estimated that 141,000 households not receiving social assistance were in abject poverty in 1994–5. Taken together with the 110,000 households then in receipt of CSSA, they concluded that about 250,000 households, or about 15.5 per cent of all households were in a state of abject poverty.

At the end of 1996 and the beginning of 1997 three further studies were released. The first two (MacPherson and Chan 1996, 1997) reported the results of a survey of 700 low income households. The survey examined the lifestyles of 'ordinary' Hong Kong households and the results gave support to the approach used to calculate the 'minimum acceptable level', which had been used in earlier assessment of the adequacy of social assistance rates. The survey found many households living below the 'minimum acceptable level' (70 per cent of the sample) and 40 per cent of all sample households were found to have income and expenditure below the prevailing rates of social assistance. Over 35 per cent of the households surveyed had per capita food expenditure which was HK$700 per month or less. The survey also showed how in very many cases it is the cost of private rented housing which is pushing households from low income into poverty. For a large number of households a high proportion of their already inadequate income was being spent on accommodation far below the standards of the meanest public housing.

The third report (MacPherson and Lo 1997) was of a detailed calculation of the number of poor people in Hong Kong. The minimum acceptable standard of living was used as the basis for an updated poverty line which included housing costs. These took household composition into account, and were calculated separately for public and private sector tenants. Applying these poverty lines to the 1995 Household Expenditure Survey data it was estimated that at least 139,500 households not in receipt of social assistance were in poverty. This was at least 375,000 people – 192,000 in private housing and 183,000 in public housing. The current social assistance (CSSA) rates are below the minimum acceptable level, and so to these numbers must be added those people in CSSA households – about 200,000. Thus the overall estimate of the number of people in poverty was 575,000, and rising.

THE FUTURE

An interesting, and potentially very important exception to the general failure of the Hong Kong government to seriously reform the social assistance scheme was the CSSA Review proposal that elderly claimants could in future be allowed to receive CSSA while resident in China. At present they can only be out of Hong Kong for half the year: the new proposal would enable them to retire to China. The administration of this scheme has yet to be worked out, although it was announced to begin in April 1997, and is potentially very difficult indeed. But this points up one fundamental and vital issue about CSSA in Hong Kong – the relationship between Hong Kong social assistance and conditions in China (Chow and Phillips 1993). Particularly outside the cities, an elderly person with a Hong Kong CSSA income would be very well off in China. The ramifications of the huge differences in income and social support levels between Hong Kong and China are enormous. The future of social assistance in Hong Kong depends above all on what the social and economic relations are between the future Hong Kong SAR and the rest of China. Most particularly this is so with Guangdong, the province bordering Hong Kong. Guangdong is experiencing very rapid economic growth, and great social change. Social security and social assistance are major issues for the region (MacPherson and Cheng 1996), and although incomes are increasing fast, conditions are still completely different from those in Hong Kong.

Although reducing levels of family support, the growing number of elderly and the anticipated influx of wives and children will be difficult for the social assistance scheme to cope with, the long-term difficulties lie elsewhere. Social assistance in Guangdong is rudimentary. In the long run the most important factor affecting social assistance in Hong Kong will be the integrity of the border, and the reality of the 'one country two systems' concept. If migration of low income households from the mainland is allowed to reach the levels typical of other very rich cities which are part of poor countries, then the social assistance scheme in Hong Kong will be in an impossible position.

CONCLUSION

One of the greatest failures of the colonial government in Hong Kong was not to implement an adequate social security programme. The adoption of means-tested social assistance, financed from general revenue, was more a product of the emphasis on minimalism as it was the product of any coherent social security planning. The recent explosion of social assistance expenditures has been the product of demographic and social changes more than changes in eligibility or benefit levels. The Hong Kong government finds itself with a massive, and growing, social assistance scheme which it certainly did not plan.

Pressure on government to do something about old age poverty resulted, eventually, in the Mandatory Provident Fund scheme, a privately-administered mandatory occupational savings programme. But this does almost nothing, even in the long run, about poverty (Dixon 1995). The impending transition of Hong Kong to the status of a Special Administrative Region of the People's Republic of China is profoundly important. The extent of social integration will determine both patterns of poverty and of social security. In March 1997 there was an editorial in the *South China Morning Post* (18 March 1997) which summed up reaction to the governments refusal to use its massive surplus for the relief of poverty:

A rich society which allows the poor in its midst to live in hunger is a society shamed. Hong Kong, with its excessive financial reserves, has over 600,000 people living below the poverty line . . . . There can be no sharper illustration of the 'unacceptable face of capitalism' than a free market which flourishes not just because of the hard work and enterprise of its people, but through the exploitation of its unskilled workers in one of the wealthiest cities in the world.

REFERENCES

Chow, N.W.S. and Phillips, D.R. (1993) 'Hong Kong and China in 1997: The Implications for Migration of Elderly People – Opportunities, Constraints, or Impetus', *Journal of Ageing and Social Policy* 5 (4): 119–36.

Dixon, J. (1995) *Mandatory Occupational Retirement Savings: Towards a Program Design Agenda for Hong Kong* (Discussion Paper 12 (2/95)), Hong Kong: Lingnan College, Centre for Public Policy Studies.

Heppell, T.S. (1974) 'Social Security and Social Welfare: a "New Look" from Hong Kong: Part Two', *Journal of Social Policy* 3 (3): 113–26.

Heppell, T.S. and Webb, P.R. (1973) 'Planning Social Welfare: the Hong Kong Experience', *International Social Work* 16 (4): 16–25.

Hong Kong Government (1967) *A Report by the Inter-Departmental Working Group to Consider Certain Aspects of Social Security*, Hong Kong: Government Printer.

—— (1995) *Hong Kong in Figures 1995*, Hong Kong: Government Printer.

—— (1996) *Report on Review of Comprehensive Social Security Assistance (CSSA) Scheme*, Hong Kong: Government Printer.

Jones, C.M. (1990) *Promoting Prosperity: The Hong Kong Way of Social Policy*, Hong Kong: Chinese University Press.

Liu, E., Yue, S.Y. and Lee, V. (1996) *Research on the Determinants for the Social Assistance Scale in Hong Kong and Selected Countries*, Hong Kong: Research and Library Services Division Legislative Council Secretariat.

Lui, T.L. and Wong, H. (1995) *Disempowerment and Empowerment – An Exploratory Study on the Low income Households in Hong Kong*, Hong Kong: Oxfam.

MacPherson, S. (1982) *Social Policy in the Third World*, Hemel Hempstead: Harvester Wheatsheaf.

—— (1994) *A Measure of Dignity: Report on the Adequacy of Public Assistance rates in Hong Kong*, Hong Kong: Hong Kong Council of Social Services.

MacPherson, S. and Chan, C.K. (1996) *Preliminary Report on a Survey of Low Income Households in Sham Shui Po*, Hong Kong: City University of Hong Kong, Department of Public and Social Administration.

—— (1997) *Housing and Poverty in Hong Kong*, Hong Kong: City University of Hong Kong, Department of Public and Social Administration.

MacPherson, S. and Cheng, J. (eds) (1996) *Economic and Social Development in South China*, Aldershot: Edward Elgar.

MacPherson, S. and Lo, O.Y. (1997) *A Measure of Poverty; Calculating the Number of People in Poverty in Hong Kong*, Hong Kong: City University of Hong Kong, Department of Public and Social Administration.

Ngan, R. (1993) 'Residualization of Social Security Protection in Hong Kong'. A paper presented at the academic forum *After retirement : Income*

Support in an Ageing Population, Hong Kong: Hong Kong Government Central Policy Unit.

—— (1996) 'Social Security and Poverty', in Chi, I. and Cheung, S.K. (eds) *Social Work in Hong Kong*, Hong Kong: Hong Kong Social Workers Association.

Sequiera, G., Howroyd, S., MacPherson, S. and Lo, O.Y. (1996) *Doing Social Research: The Poverty Project in Hong Kong*, Hong Kong: Asia Pacific Social Development Research Centre.

Wong, H and Chua H.W. (1996) *Household Expenditure Patterns of Low Income Households, Hong Kong*, Hong Kong: Hong Kong Council of Social Services.

Chapter 5

Ireland

Tim Callan and Brian Nolan

Much attention has been given in Ireland, as in many other countries, to the increase in average living standards made possible by economic growth and development. In the 1960s the slogan that 'a rising tide lifts all boats' was used to justify a very strong focus on growth. But concerns about the distribution of the benefits of growth, the persistence of high rates of unemployment, and the adequacy of incomes for individuals dependent on the social welfare system re-emerged particularly strongly during the 1980s and 1990s.

Measurement of poverty in Ireland has, until relatively recently, been hampered by the lack of the necessary micro-level data on individual and household incomes. Data are now available, however, for selected years spanning the 1973 to 1994 period. This chapter summarises very briefly the main results of a broad programme of research on poverty measurement, dealing with this period; outlines the response of social welfare and other policies in tackling the poverty problem; and highlights the key issues in looking to the future (see also Nolan and Callan 1994; Callan *et al*. 1996). First, however, we provide a brief overview of the development of Ireland as an independent economy and society, to assist the reader in comparing the profile of poverty and anti-poverty policy in Ireland with those for other countries.

IRELAND: *A TOUR D'HORIZON*

The Republic of Ireland emerged as an independent entity in 1922, the date of the treaty establishing the Irish Free State as an independent member of the British Commonwealth – an important watershed in the long and complex relationship between Ireland

and the United Kingdom (UK), their nearest neighbour and former colonial power. Moves towards greater independence culminated in the declaration of a republic in 1947 (for an analysis of poverty in Northern Ireland see Borooah and McGregor 1991; for a comparison of the level and composition of poverty in the Republic of Ireland and Northern Ireland, see Heaton *et al.* 1991). The population of Ireland now stands at about 3.6 million, up from its nadir of about 2.8 million in 1961. The population of the same land area stood at about 6.5 million prior to the Great Famine of 1845–50, and was reduced by deaths and emigration to 5.1 million in 1851 (Ireland 1995).

Poverty in Ireland today is different from poverty in developing countries, where absolute measures focused on the minimum needed for survival may be of central importance; and different from poverty in Ireland in earlier years – dramatically different from its meaning at the time of the Great Famine in the 1840s. However, an understanding of contemporary Irish society requires some knowledge of its history as well as of its current demographic, social and economic structure (for an account of economic and social development in pre- and post-famine Ireland, see O'Grada 1994)

At independence, Gross Domestic Product (GDP) per capita stood at about 55 per cent of the UK level (Kennedy *et al.* 1988) which placed it roughly mid-way in the ranking of European countries. By the 1980s it had reached about two-thirds of the UK level; but as the UK had experienced slow growth relative to other Western European countries, Ireland had fallen to a much lower place in the output rankings. Rapid growth over much of the past decade means that in the mid-1990s, Ireland's GDP per capita is close to that of the UK and the average for the European Union (EU). It should be noted that profit repatriation by multinational companies and other factors make Gross National Product (GNP) in Ireland lower than GDP, by a margin greater than in most other countries. However, the GDP-based comparisons serve to illustrate the impact of recent rapid growth on Ireland's position within Europe.

Since independence, industry and latterly services have grown in importance, while the share of agriculture in output and employment has declined. Industrialisation proceeded at first under the shelter of protection, but a shift to outward looking policies began in the 1950s, as the limits of protection became clear, with poor economic performance and renewed emigration. Trade with the UK was liberalised under a bilateral agreement in 1966, and in 1973

Ireland, along with the UK, joined the European Economic Community (EEC).

Membership of the EEC has had a substantial impact on subsequent economic development. Agriculture benefited from the EEC's Common Agricultural Policy, while foreign direct investment was boosted as Ireland became a European base for firms from the US and elsewhere. The oil-price shocks in 1973 and 1979, together with the associated international recessions, had a serious impact on growth and particularly on unemployment. The policy response included pump-priming measures which had limited effects on employment, given the openness of the economy. The more lasting effect of these policies was on the public finances, with current budget deficits leading to a substantial debt burden. The debt problem was brought under control in the late 1980s and early 1990s, with tax revenues rising as the economy moved onto a path of stronger growth. The completion of the Single European Market, and financial assistance under EU financed programme (the 'cohesion' measures, structural funds and the Community Support Framework, associated with the further integration of the economies of EU countries) have contributed to this growth, which has seen Ireland outperform most of its EU partners. Investment by multinational companies is still strong, with a particularly strong representation in chemicals, pharmaceuticals, computers and other high technology sectors.

Ireland's demographic experience in the twentieth century has been rather different from the international norm. Fertility declined rather slowly up to the 1970s, with more rapid declines elsewhere leaving Ireland as an increasingly anomalous example of persistent high fertility. A continuing pattern of emigration meant that population declined for most of this period. In more recent years, however, there have been dramatic demographic changes, with declines in fertility, emigration and immigration (mostly return migration) roughly in balance, and modest increases in population. Emigration in the economically active age groups during the 1950s, coupled with high fertility, had led to a high dependency ratio. This has now declined, and is set to decline further in future years.

MEASURING POVERTY

Measures of poverty in Ireland have, as in most developed countries, concentrated on defining a poverty line in terms of income, and regarding those with incomes below the line as poor. A number of different approaches have been applied (see Callan and Nolan 1991; Nolan and Callan 1994). None of these approaches can avoid the arbitrary element of judgement in establishing an income cut-off. There is a great deal of uncertainty and disagreement over the location of the poverty line; and life is not very different for those with incomes just above or just below any such line. One practical method of poverty measurement which can take account of these facts is the relative income poverty line approach, which derives poverty line incomes as fixed proportions of average incomes, adjusted for family size and composition using equivalence scales. (The equivalence scale used in the measures reported here – and used in Figures 5.1 and 5.2 – is 1 for the first adult in a household, 0.66 for other adults, and 0.33 for children aged under 14. We focus mainly on results which are robust with respect to the equivalence scale; results which are sensitive to the scale used are noted in the text.) A cut-off of half average income is most commonly used, but profiles of poverty at alternative cut-offs such as 40 per cent and 60 per cent of average income can also be examined, and help to identify conclusions which are robust with respect to the level of the poverty cut-off. A further advantage of this approach is that it requires relatively straightforward information on income and household composition, which is available for many countries, and, in the Irish case, for each of the years 1973, 1980, 1987 and 1994. More detailed data relevant to poverty are available for Ireland for 1987 and 1994, from the Economic and Social Research Institute (ESRI) household surveys in those years, which have allowed alternative measures of poverty to be implemented.

Income-based poverty lines can be seen as focusing wholly on the 'resources' element of the Townsend definition. But as Ringen (1988) points out, low income is not a reliable measure of *exclusion* arising from lack of resources. Nolan and Whelan (1996) and Callan, Nolan and Whelan (1993) argue that a more reliable measure of exclusion due to lack of resources can be constructed given suitable direct information on indicators of deprivation – items generally regarded as necessities, which individuals or families must do without because they 'cannot afford' them. This approach combines information on income and on indicators of deprivation to provide an alternative identification of those who are poor.

Turning to the *aggregation* issue, we find that the head count ratio – the proportion of individuals or families who are identified as poor – is still the most widely used measure of poverty, despite its well known defects. But alternative measures which take into account the depth and distribution of poverty have been developed for income-based measures of poverty. In this chapter we present results based on Foster, Greer and Thorbecke's (1984) income gap ratio – a measure which combines information on the extent and depth of poverty – and their depth and distribution sensitive measure, which gives particular weight to those on the lowest incomes.

The household is the unit of analysis most commonly employed in studies of poverty. Implicitly this treats all members of a household as having a common standard of living. This assumption may be inappropriate for some households. Considerable efforts were made – including the collection of detailed data on household's allocation systems – to investigate the issues of allocation of resources within households and families (Rottman 1994). The results of this study, and of an alternative investigation of differences in living standards between husbands and wives (Cantillon and Nolan, forthcoming 1998), while not conclusive, do not suggest that a substantial reservoir of hidden poverty exists at sub-household level in Ireland. Thus, in what follows, we focus on the household level of analysis as is customary in most countries. However, we focus particularly on measures which count the number of individuals in poor households, rather than simply counting the number or proportion of households in poverty. The average income measure is obtained by taking the mean of income per adult equivalent over all households. While the alternative of taking mean income per adult equivalent over all individuals is of interest (and is used, for example, in the UK's statistics on *Households Below Average Income*), comparability with analyses for the years 1973 and 1980 requires that we adopt the 'average over households' instead.

In undertaking comparisons over time a key issue is how the poverty standard should be up-rated. Standards constructed to represent a particular standard of living 'in real terms' are of value – for example, in establishing whether or not the poor have benefited from a period of economic growth – but over any prolonged period where real incomes are rising they will lose contact with the reality of life in the society, and what it means to be poor in that society. The relative income poverty line approach adopted here implicitly up-rates the poverty line in line with average incomes.

From a cross-country point of view the key implication of

measures based on poverty as a proportion of average income is that the poverty line for a rich country is much higher than that for a poor country. In making comparisons with other country studies in this volume, it should be borne in mind that Ireland ranks as one of the high-income countries in the World Bank's (1996) classification, with GNP per capita at US$13,000 in 1993 terms – about the same level as New Zealand, Spain or Israel.

THE INCIDENCE OF POVERTY

We focus initially on results from the relative income poverty line approach, based on a measure of current disposable income. (For farmers and the self-employed the income figures refer to a full year, as sub-annual variation in receipts and expenditure can be considerable.) We note briefly some results applying the relative income approach to alternative measures of resources, and then discuss the incidence of poverty obtained by combining measures of income and deprivation.

The head count ratios (Figure 5.1) show that the incidence of poverty is very sensitive to the level of the poverty line. In 1994, about 22 per cent of persons are found to have incomes below half the average, with about seven per cent having incomes below 40 per cent of the average, and close to 35 per cent having incomes below the 60 per cent cut-off. Since there is no strong *a priori* reason to choose any one of these lines as 'the' indicator of poverty, it is useful to put the income levels corresponding to these lines into perspective. In 1987, the 40 per cent cut-off corresponded roughly to the lowest rates of social welfare payment (for short-term social assistance under the Supplementary Welfare Allowance scheme – the Irish 'safety net' scheme – and short-term means-tested benefits to the unemployed); the 50 per cent cut-off coincided roughly with the payment rate for Unemployment Benefit (paid to unemployed workers covered by social insurance); while the 60 per cent cut-off lay between the means-tested and insurance-based payments to old age pensioners. By 1994, dispersion in social welfare payment rates had been reduced through faster than average increases for schemes with the lowest payments. Thus, the 40 per cent cut-off fell below the minimum social welfare payment, while the 50 per cent cut-off was somewhat above it. The 60 per cent cut-off in 1994 was above the Old Age Contributory Pension paid by the social security system.

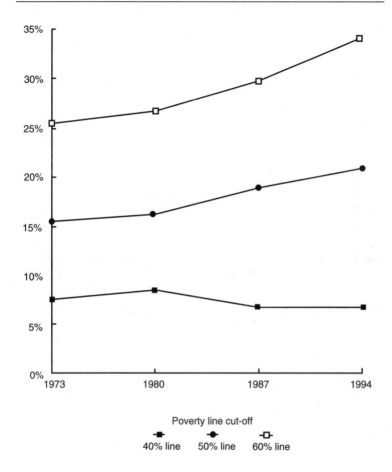

Figure 5.1 Proportion of individuals below relative income poverty
lines: 1973–94

Note: Poverty line cut-off per cent uses equivalence scale (1 for the first adult,
0.66 for other adults and 0.33 for children)

Trends in the head count ratio over time also vary somewhat
with the level of the poverty line, though far less dramatically.
Between 1973 and 1994, the head count ratio falls slightly at the
40 per cent relative income poverty line, but rises by about 5
percentage points for the poverty line at half average income, and
by about 7 percentage points at the 60 per cent line.

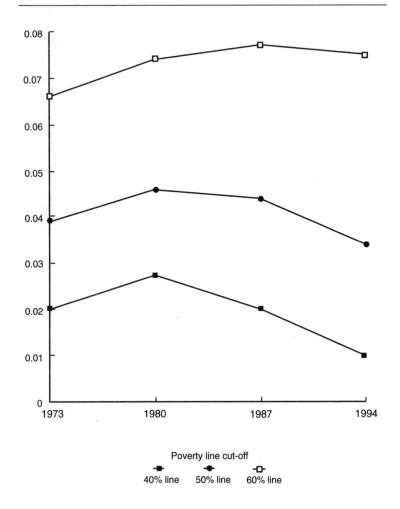

Figure 5.2 Per capita income gaps at alternative relative income
            poverty lines: 1973–94

Note: Poverty line cut-off per cent uses equivalence scale (1 for the first adult,
        0.66 for other adults and 0.33 for children)

Measures which take into account the depth, as well as the extent
of income poverty, tell a rather different story. The *per capita income
gap* (as measured by P_2 in Foster *et al.* (1984)), measures the aggregate of the income gaps of those below the poverty line, expressed as

a proportion of the poverty line, divided by the total population. Thus it takes into account the number of people falling below the line, and the depth of their poverty. It would reach a maximum, equal to the head count ratio, if each poor person had a zero income; and would be close to zero if each poor person fell *just below* the poverty line. These indicators show a rise in poverty between 1973 and 1980, but a fall at the 40 per cent and 50 per cent cut-offs in each of the later sub-periods (1980–7 and 1987–94). Over the full period, the per capita income gap shows a fall in poverty at the 40 per cent and 50 per cent relative income lines, with a small increase at the 60 per cent line. The *depth- and distribution-sensitive index* of poverty proposed by Foster, Greer and Thorbecke (1984) gives greatest weight to the 'poorest of the poor' in income terms. For Ireland, this measure shows a fall in poverty at each of the relative income cut-offs between 1973 and 1987, including the 60 per cent relative income line.

In our brief discussion of measures of poverty, we noted that measures combining information on income and indicators of deprivation had been developed to assist in identifying those who are most clearly excluded from ordinary living patterns by lack of resources. These measures are available for 1987 and 1994, from two surveys conducted by the ESRI: the 1987 Survey of Income Distribution, Poverty and Usage of State Services, and the 1994 *Living in Ireland Survey*, which forms part of the European Community Household Panel managed by Eurostat. A set of eight items and activities was identified from a more extensive list as particularly useful. The items include a substantial meal every day, new rather than second-hand clothes, and a meal with meat, chicken or fish every other day. Essentially the same deprivation indicators were used in 1987 and 1994 – a procedure which can be seen as somewhat conservative, in that what counts as a necessity can be expected to change over time. These items are widely regarded as possessed or engaged in by a majority of the population, and are found to 'cluster together' in a factor analysis of the larger set of items. An 'enforced lack' of any one of these eight basic items (that is, if the household has to do without the item because, in the view of the respondent, they cannot afford it) is treated as an indicator of underlying generalised deprivation. A measure of poverty combining income and deprivation information is obtained by regarding a household as poor if its income falls below the 60 per cent relative income poverty line and it is experiencing basic deprivation (for more details on the rationale for this approach, its implementation, and its implications see Nolan and Whelan 1996.)

In 1987, more than half of those falling below the 60 per cent relative income line were found to be suffering from an enforced lack of one or more of the basic items. Thus, about 16 per cent of all households were found to be below the income threshold and experiencing basic deprivation. By 1994, this figure had fallen marginally, to just under 15 per cent: a rise in the proportion of households found below the income threshold was offset by the fact that less than half of these households were now found to be experiencing basic deprivation.

WHO ARE THE POOR?

Who are the poor households? This is a key policy question. The answers vary over time, and appropriate policy responses must also shift in response to these changes. In this section we show how the characteristics of those identified as poor by relative income poverty lines have changed over time in Ireland, and how an alternative definition of poverty – using information on deprivation indicators as well as income – can affect the profile of the poverty population.

In describing the characteristics of the poverty population and comparing them with the general population we make use of two perspectives. We look at the *incidence* of poverty for particular groups (that is, the *proportion of all those in poverty* who belong to that group). We also consider the *risk* of poverty for the group (that is, the *proportion of that group* which falls below the relevant income standard).

Developments during the 1973 to 1987 and the 1987 to 1994 sub-periods were somewhat different, so we consider them in turn. Tables 5.1 and 5.2 shows the incidence and risk of poverty for each year.

During the 1973 to 1987 sub-period, the key features were a rise in the proportion of poor households which were headed by an unemployed person, and a fall in the proportion headed by the elderly – a group which included many women classified as in 'home duties' as well as men and women classified as retired. In 1973, households headed by a person who was retired or in home duties formed about 42 per cent of the population of households below half average income; by 1987, this figure had fallen to around 15 per cent. At the same time, the proportion of poor households headed by an unemployed person rose from just under 10 per cent

Table 5.1 Composition of households below half average income by labour force status of household head

	Households below half average income (%)				Total households in sample (%)			
	1973	1980	1987	1994	1973	1980	1987	1994
Labour force status								
Employee	9.0	10.3	8.2	6.2	42.4	47.1	38.6	37.5
Self-employed	3.6	3.5	4.8	6.7	6.5	6.8	7.5	8.5
Farmer	26.0	25.9	23.7	8.9	22.4	16.1	11.7	8.1
Unemployed	9.6	14.7	37.4	32.6	2.9	3.9	10.6	10.2
Ill/disabled	10.2	9.3	11.1	9.5	4.5	3.3	6.0	4.0
Retired	17.0	18.9	8.1	10.5	10.6	13.7	14.5	18.3
Home duties	24.6	17.4	6.7	25.5	10.7	9.1	11.1	13.5
Total	100.0	100.0	100.0	100.0	100.0	100.0	100.0	100.0

Table 5.2 Risks (%) of relative poverty (at half average income) classified by labour force status of head of household: 1973–94

	Below line (%)			
	1973	1980	1987	1994
Labour force status				
Employee	3.9	3.7	3.5	3.1
Self-employed	10.1	8.6	10.5	14.7
Farmer	21.2	27.0	32.8	20.4
Unemployed	61.9	63.1	57.2	59.4
Ill/disabled	42.8	48.2	33.7	44.5
Retired	29.5	23.3	9.1	10.6
Home duties	42.2	32.2	9.8	34.9
Total	18.3	16.8	16.3	18.5

to 37 per cent. The proportion of low income households headed by a farmer was roughly constant, at about 25 per cent: an increased risk of poverty for farmers, relative to the general population offset the secular decline in the numbers working as farmers over this sub-period. It must be stressed, however, that the farm income figure used in the 1987 survey was for 1986 – the latest available year – but one which was the nadir of farm incomes during the 1980s.

An alternative, purely demographic perspective confirms that households headed by an elderly person were at particularly high risk of poverty in 1973. The risk of poverty was quite high for the unemployed, but in 1973 they formed a much smaller proportion of the population than in later years. The fall in the risk of relative poverty for those who are retired is mainly due to increased and improved coverage by occupational pension schemes, and to improved coverage and increased rates of payments for social welfare schemes dealing with the elderly – as will be seen in the next section.

The growing share of the poverty population made up of house-holds headed by an unemployed person reflects largely the general rise in unemployment over the period, rather than a rise in the risk of poverty for those who are unemployed. This shift in the composi-tion of the poverty population carries with it an increased risk of poverty for families at a stage in the life-cycle when there are depen-dent children. Thus, the risk of income poverty for children (at the half of average income standard) has almost doubled – from 16 per cent in 1973 to 29 per cent in 1994 – while the risk for adults has risen much less (from 15 to 18 per cent).

Developments in the 1987 to 1994 period have been somewhat different. Unemployment remains the major cause of poverty, and the risk of income poverty for the retired remains well below average. But the risk of income poverty for women in home duties – mostly elderly and/or widowed – has risen sharply in this sub-period. Figures for 1994 show a fall in the risk of poverty for farm households, to a level just below the 1973 rate, and a much smaller incidence of farm households in the poverty population.

At a higher income cut-off (the 60 per cent relative poverty line), we find that the pattern of risk remains rather similar. The highest risk is for the unemployed, with households headed by an employee or self-employed person facing a below average risk. The main change in the pattern is that at the higher poverty line, the risk for the ill/disabled and those in home duties rises sharply relative to the average, to levels close to those for the unemployed. To a large extent this reflects the pattern of social welfare rates, which will be discussed in the next section.

For 1987 and 1994, it is possible to use the combined income/deprivation indicator approach to identify those households most clearly excluded from ordinary living standards through lack of resources. This identifies rather fewer farmers and self-employed as 'poor' than the income-based measure. This difference was particularly marked in 1987, when farm incomes were particularly low, and may not have corresponded with farm households longer-term command over resources. But even in 1994, this difference is a notable feature of the comparison between income-based poverty measures (with 19 per cent of households below half average income) and the combined income-deprivation indicator approach (with 15 per cent of households below 60 per cent of average income and suffering enforced lack of a basic necessity). A common core of about nine per cent of households were identified as poor under both of these measures, with a further 10 per cent of households falling below half average income, or a further 7 per cent of households falling below 60 per cent income standard and suffering basic deprivation.

SOCIAL SECURITY RESPONSES TO POVERTY

When Ireland gained independence in 1922, it inherited a social security system essentially identical to that of the UK at that time. (In line with usage elsewhere in this volume, we use the term social security to cover both social insurance and social assistance; in Ireland the term social welfare is used to cover both elements.) This included an Old Age Pension, workmen's compensation, some elements of National Insurance, and the 'Poor Law' system. Many later developments also mirrored those in the UK, though in more recent years the Irish and UK systems have tended to diverge in a number of respects – with Irish rates of payment now quite often somewhat above UK rates (relative to average income, or, in some cases, in absolute terms) though still somewhat below average EU levels (Callan and Sutherland 1997).

The broad structure of the social security system during the 1973 to 1994 period comprised a system of social insurance – with contributions from employers, employees and the state financing contributory benefits – and a system of social assistance – with means-tested payments also provided for many of the same contingencies (old age, unemployment) as for the contributory schemes. A universal child benefit payment was introduced as early as 1944, but was, until recently, quite low in comparison to the payments made as 'child dependent additions' to recipients of most social security schemes (contributory and non-contributory). Despite recent increases, the rate of child benefit is about one-third of the *total* payment (comprising child benefit and a 'child dependent addition') received in respect of children by most social security beneficiaries.

A new social assistance scheme, the Supplementary Welfare Allowance, was established in 1975 to provide a standard national income 'safety net' replacing the old 'home assistance' service (which varied across local authority jurisdictions). The payment rate for the new scheme is rate equal to that for short-term unemployment assistance. Social insurance contributions were made pay-related in 1979. A number of smaller schemes were put in place during the 1960s and early 1970s – including provision for deserted wives and lone parents, which has since grown rapidly in importance.

One approach towards gauging the overall impact of the social security system in reducing poverty is that provided by Beckerman (1979). It is built around the concept of pre-transfer income, defined simply as actual income less public transfers. He defines *poverty reduction efficiency* as the proportion of social security expenditure which goes towards reducing the pre-transfer aggregate poverty gap (the sum of all the gaps between the pre-transfer incomes of those below a poverty standard, and the standard itself). The *poverty reduction effectiveness* of the system is the proportion of the pre-transfer aggregate poverty gap which is reduced by transfers.

Obviously the poverty reduction efficiency and effectiveness of the system will depend *inter alia* on the level of the poverty standard chosen, as well as on the structure of pre-transfer poverty and the social security system itself. For this reason, it is of interest to examine measures of poverty reduction effectiveness and efficiency at a range of income poverty lines. While the social security system operates at a number of levels, the narrower family unit is a good proxy for the benefit unit. Analysis undertaken at that level (using 1987 data) suggests that between 54 and 77 per cent of transfers go towards poverty reduction at income standards from 40 per cent to 60 per cent of average income; and that between 80 and 70 per cent of the pre-transfer poverty gap at these income standards is eliminated by transfers. A similar pattern of results is found at household level, although at lower levels of effectiveness and efficiency.

These results are heavily influenced by differences in payment rates within the social security system. Payment rates in 1987 varied considerably between contributory and non-contributory schemes, and between the elderly, widows and the unemployed. The lowest rates of payment were close to the 40 per cent relative income line, while the highest rates were close to the 60 per cent relative income standard. Lower efficiency at the lowest poverty line largely reflects the fact that payment rates for many schemes were sufficient, even if the recipients had no other income, to raise incomes above that poverty standard. Lower effectiveness at the highest relative poverty line reflects, in turn, the fact that several important schemes had a rate of payment well below that level.

International comparisons of analyses of this type are dogged by problems of comparability. However, the Irish data and analysis formed part of a harmonised international project on measurement of poverty and the effectiveness of social security in a number of European countries (Deleeck *et al.* 1992). This suggests that the Irish social security system is markedly more 'efficient', in the Beckerman sense, than those of the Benelux countries over a wide range of poverty lines. The Irish system is, however, somewhat less effective. The size of the pre-transfer poverty gap is relatively large in Ireland: it forms over 15 per cent of aggregate household income, as against about 10 per cent in the Netherlands. This means that a given proportion of national income devoted to social security, at any given level of efficiency, will tend to be less effective in Ireland than in countries such as Belgium and the Netherlands, with a lower pre-transfer poverty gap.

The profile of poverty in 1973 showed the elderly to be a high risk group, forming a substantial proportion of all households in poverty. Partly in response to this finding, rates of payment for Old Age Contributory and Non-Contributory Pensions increased quite rapidly during the late 1970s and early 1980s. This, taken together with the rise in the coverage of occupational pensions, contributed to a substantial improvement in the income position of the elderly relative to other groups in the period to 1987.

Social security policy between 1987 and 1994 was heavily influenced by the findings of the Commission on Social Welfare (Ireland, CSW 1985), which focused particular attention on the inadequacy of the lowest payment rates and set an adequacy standard approximating the higher rates of payment. (For a recent review of the issues raised by the Commission's findings, see Callan *et al.* 1996.) Thus, while rates for the highest paid schemes were increased only marginally ahead of the rate of price inflation, special increases in the rates of payment for the lowest paid schemes – Unemployment Assistance and the safety net of Supplementary Welfare Allowance – were introduced. This process led to a considerable reduction in the dispersion of payment rates across social security schemes.

The structure of social security payments, with additions for adult and child dependants, led to concerns about the financial incentives to work faced by welfare recipients with many dependants. In its most severe form this became known as the 'unemployment trap', in which an individual had little or no financial incentive to take up employment. By the early 1980s, these concerns led to the introduction of the Family Income Supplement, paid to individuals whose income from employment was low relative to their family size. While this structure offered some improvement in the financial incentive to take up (or remain in) employment (an improvement on the 'unemployment trap') it contributed to a new 'poverty trap', whereby an increase in gross earnings triggered a combination of benefit reductions and tax increases which could leave an individual worse off, or no better off, than before the earnings increase. In addition, the Family Income Supplement scheme suffered from a continuing problem of low take-up, with many of those eligible not actually obtaining the benefit: this reduces its effectiveness in maintaining financial incentives to work. These issues were reconsidered by an Expert Working Group on the Integration of the Income Tax and Social Welfare Systems (Ireland, Expert Group 1996), which pointed to a combination of measures – including cuts in income taxes and social insurance contributions and a restructuring of child income support – as having the potential to improve this situation.

ANTI-POVERTY PROGRAMMES

For many years, the evolution of policy could be interpreted as viewing poverty as a 'social welfare issue' – to be tackled by increased payment rates, or new schemes to cover groups with a high risk of poverty – such as the small, but growing numbers of lone parents. The fact that the poverty problem was particularly severe for the elderly contributed to the apparent strength of this view. Increases in social security pensions were seen as an effective way of targeting resources to those in need, with relatively minor impact on financial incentives to work for most of those seeking employment.

This strategy was quite effective in combating poverty among the elderly, a group which dominated the poverty population in 1973. But the emergence and persistence of high rates of unemployment made such a strategy difficult, if not impossible, to maintain in the 1980s and 1990s. During this period, the composition of poverty shifted substantially, with unemployment now seen as the main cause of poverty. Correspondingly, anti-poverty policy is now viewed in much wider terms. This has been explicitly recognised in a number of ways – from the setting up of a state-funded organisation (the Combat Poverty Agency, set up in 1986, with a wide-ranging brief, including policy advice, project support and innovation, research and public education) to the initiation of a process leading to a National Anti-Poverty Strategy (NAPS).

The recent review of anti-poverty policy by the Inter-departmental Policy Committee on the National Anti-Poverty Strategy in 1995 outlines the main areas of policy seen as contributing to the fight against poverty. This includes general economic policy, aimed at maximising the growth in employment; labour market programmes, aimed at ensuring that the long-term unemployed and other disadvantaged groups can break the cycle of deprivation by obtaining a job; education and training programmes, aimed at preventing additions to the stock of long-term unemployed, or improving the skills of those who are long-term unemployed; community development initiatives, aimed at improving the economy and/or quality of life in particular areas; and a number of initiatives in the areas of health and housing.

Evaluation of anti-poverty programmes

The overall evaluation of anti-poverty policy has been greatly hampered by the lack of regular up-to-date data of the type needed to construct measures of poverty. The main data sources which have this capability have been the Central Statistics Office's Household Budget Survey, conducted at seven-yearly intervals since 1973; the ESRI's 1987 survey, and the ongoing *Living in Ireland* panel survey, conducted by the ESRI. This has meant that monitoring of poverty outcomes has been restricted to seven-yearly intervals. The new panel survey offers some scope for more regular monitoring of developments.

Despite these difficulties in monitoring overall developments, the impact of some anti-poverty programmes have been evaluated – sometimes in quite intensive fashion. Here we focus on the evaluation of three main types of policy: tax-transfer policies, labour market and training interventions, and community development initiatives.

We described earlier some results concerning the overall impact of social security expenditures on poverty, arising from the Beckerman (1979) framework. While this framework is helpful in assessing the overall anti-poverty impact of the welfare system, it does not take account of behavioural responses to the existence of benefits and the taxes required to finance them. An alternative approach, which allows the exploration of *changes* to tax and transfer policies, including first-round effects on incomes and financial incentives to work, is provided by tax-benefit modelling. A microsimulation model of the Irish tax and social security systems has been developed at the ESRI (Callan *et al.* 1996) and has been applied in examining the impact of alternative tax and welfare policy changes on poverty, the distribution of income and the financial incentive to work facing those in employment, unemployed or not in the labour force. Model-based analyses were used by the Expert Working Group on the Integration of the Income Tax and Social Welfare Systems (Ireland, Expert Group 1996) to explore alternative forms of radical reform based on the idea of a 'basic income', and alternative options for the reform of child income support, including a 'basic income for children', and an increased, but taxable, child benefit payment.

Breen (1994) emphasises that labour market interventions can be aimed either at increasing the total numbers employed, or at ensuring that employers hire from groups who would otherwise experience continuing or long-term unemployment. Marginal employment subsidies could be aimed at encouraging hires that would otherwise not take place (increasing the numbers employed); but conditions attached to job subsidies may also be used to encourage the hiring of particular groups identified as having difficulty competing in the labour market. Thus the distribution of employment (and conversely, of unemployment) may be a concern of anti-poverty policy as well as its total level.

Breen examined the overall impact of a number of employment schemes, ranging from permanent job creation in existing firms, to assistance in starting new firms and temporary job creation. His conclusion is that such schemes have very little impact on overall employment and unemployment levels, for a number of reasons – including 'dead-weight' – exchequer payments that have no economic effect – arising from hires that employers would have made even in the absence of the intervention. The main exception to this is direct job creation by the government, with the magnitude of the effect on poverty being limited by the numbers employed on such schemes, the fact that they are temporary in nature, and the relatively low wage rates paid on the schemes. As regards targeting of labour market interventions to increase the probability of employment for those in poverty, Breen notes that difficulties in persuading employers to hire from the stock of long-term unemployed may have limited this equity effect of targeted programmes. Overall, then, it would seem that the impact of labour market interventions on poverty as assessed by Breen (1994) is quite limited.

A number of strands have led to the development of community or area based approaches to the combating of poverty. These include the pilot schemes introduced under the EU's three Programmes to Combat Poverty; the 'bottom-up' evolution of community organisations aimed at improving economic, social and personal development within their own areas; and increasing recognition of the valuable contribution made by such efforts at national level. Expenditure on these schemes has been relatively modest, and so has their direct impact, though a gradual extension to a wider geographic coverage has been taking place and important lessons can be learnt from experience so far. Such area-based approaches can clearly make a significant contribution in harnessing the energies of local communities and combating powerlessness and exclusion. The limitations of such strategies must also be recognised: it is not realistic to expect local area-based initiatives to deal with a national unemployment problem, and they have to be seen as only one element in a strategic response to poverty. In any case, although particular areas with very high unemployment and poverty rates clearly face very special challenges, most of the unemployed and most poor people are not concentrated in those areas (Nolan et al. 1994).

Where 'black spots' of pronounced urban disadvantage do exist they are for the most part in public housing, and state housing policy must take some of the blame. Large clusters of public housing in the major cities were originally built for rental, but in the 1980s – following the UK – some of this housing stock was sold to tenants on very attractive terms. This tended to exacerbate the divide between the clusters sold to households with income from work, and those remaining in public ownership where the proportion unemployed or depending on social security for other reasons, and the proportion below conventional relative poverty lines, rose (Nolan *et al.* 1997; Fahey and Watson 1995). With little new construction of public housing in recent years, housing policy and particularly the provision of assistance with housing costs for the poor is currently in a state of flux.

Some anti-poverty policy initiatives, including some undertaken on a pilot basis and/or at relatively low cost, have been investigated very intensively. Not all public expenditures, however, have been subjected to equally searching tests of their effectiveness in attaining their intended goals. Breen (1994) stresses, for example, that expenditure on labour market interventions for schemes such as marginal employment subsidies have been rigorously evaluated, but the employment impact of much greater expenditures (and tax breaks), also aimed at increasing employment, have not been subjected to the same sort of comprehensive evaluation. If rational choices are to be made about the appropriate use of resources to combat poverty and increase employment, 'a broader view must be taken in which all forms of Government expenditure in pursuit of job creation are audited for their effects on poverty and evaluated in a comparable and comprehensive manner' (Breen 1994: 292).

FUTURE PROSPECTS AND STRATEGIES

Ireland has seen strong economic growth over much of the past decade. Employment has begun to pick up strongly, particularly in the recent past. But a substantial problem of unemployment, and particularly long-term unemployment, remains.

In the near future, policy will be shaped to a great extent by the recent agreement between the government and social partners (employers, trade unions, farm organisations and others – including, for the first time, some representatives of the unemployed and disabled). This agreement (*Partnership 2000 for Inclusion, Employment and Competitiveness*) consists of a three-and-a-half year programme covering pay, tax, social security and a wide range of other government policies. It includes a set of measures under the heading of 'promoting greater social inclusion' which deal very directly with the problems of poverty and 'social exclusion' – defined in the document as 'cumulative marginalisation: from production (unemployment), from consumption (income poverty), from social networks (community, family and neighbours), from decision-making and from an adequate quality of life'.

The main features of the social inclusion package are:

• the adoption of a National Anti-Poverty Strategy in early 1997, which involves the setting of objectives and strategies to be pursued in tackling unemployment, educational disadvantage, income adequacy and the regeneration of disadvantaged urban communities with concentrations of poverty, and in tackling of poverty in rural areas; and new institutional mechanisms designed to produce a co-ordinated approach across government departments;
• an expansion of targeted employment and training measures, and further development of public employment services;
• an expansion of targeted programmes aimed at breaking the cycle of educational disadvantage;
• real increases in social security payments sufficient to reach – in real terms, although not in relative terms – the standards identified by the Commission on Social Welfare (1985); and
• a number of specific commitments regarding anti-poverty actions at local level, including both urban and rural areas.

The medium-term macroeconomic prospects for the Irish economy appear bright. A key task for research is to explain how recent growth, and associated policy developments, have affected the extent, depth and nature of poverty. This knowledge can be expected to contribute to the development of anti-poverty strategy in the future.

ACKNOWLEDGEMENTS

This chapter has drawn on the 1994 wave of the *Living in Ireland Survey*, the Irish element of the European Community Household Panel. Brendan Whelan and James Williams of the ESRI's Survey Unit were responsible for the survey design, data collection and database creation.

Thanks are also due to Brendan Whelan and Damian Hannan for initiating the ESRI's 1987 Survey of Income Distribution, Poverty and Usage of State Services, which provided the springboard for much of the work on poverty measurement in Ireland; and to Chris Whelan for his collaboration on the programme of work on poverty measurement summarised here.

REFERENCES

Beckerman, W. (1979) 'The Impact of Income Maintenance Payments on Poverty in Britain', *Economic Journal* 89 (2): 261–79.

Borooah, V. and McGregor, P. (1991) 'The Measurement and Decomposition of Poverty: An Analysis Based on the 1985 Family Expenditure Survey For Northern Ireland', *Manchester School*.

Breen, R. (1994) 'Poverty and Labour Market Measures', in Nolan, B. and Callan, T. (eds) *Poverty And Policy In Ireland*, Dublin: Gill and Macmillan.

Callan, T. and Nolan, B. (1991) 'Concepts of Poverty and the Poverty Line', *Journal of Economic Surveys* 5 (3): 243–61.

Callan, T., Nolan, B., Whelan, B.J., Whelan, C.T. and Williams, J. (1996) *Poverty in the 1990s: Evidence from the Living in Ireland Survey*, Dublin: Oak Tree Press.

Callan, T., Nolan, B. and Whelan, C.T. (1993) 'Resources, Deprivation and the Measurement of Poverty', *Journal of Social Policy* 22 (2): 141–72.

—— (1996) *A Review of the Commission on Social Welfare's Minimum Adequate Income* (Policy Research Series Number 29), Dublin: The Economic And Social Research Institute.

Callan, T., O'Donoghue, C. and O'Neill, C. (1996) *SWITCH: The ESRI Tax-Benefit Model*, Dublin: The Economic and Social Research Institute.

Callan, T. and Sutherland, H. (1997) 'Income Supports in Ireland and the UK' in Callan, T. (ed.) *Income Support and Work Incentives: Ireland and the UK* (Institute Policy Research Series Paper No. 30), Dublin: The Economic and Social Research Institute.

Cantillon, S. and Nolan, B. (1998) 'Are Married Women more Deprived than their Husbands?', *Journal of Social Policy*, forthcoming.

Deleeck, H., van den Bosch, K. and Lathouwer, L. (eds) (1992) *Poverty and the Adequacy of Social Security in the EC: A Comparative Analysis*, Aldershot: Avebury.

Fahey, T. and Watson, D. (1995) *An Analysis of Housing Need* (General Research Series Paper No. 168), Dublin: The Economic and Social Research Institute.

Foster, J.E., Greer, J. and Thorbecke, E. (1984) 'A Class of Decomposable Poverty Measures', *Econometrica* 52 (4): 761–6.

Heaton, N., Callan, T., Borooah, V. and Nolan, B. (1991) 'Poverty in the "North" and "South" of Ireland' (*Mimeo*), Jordanstown: University of Ulster at Jordanstown.

Ireland, Commission on Social Welfare (CSW) (1985) *Report of the Commission on Social Welfare*, Dublin: Stationery Office.

Ireland (1995) *Facts About Ireland*, Dublin: Department of Foreign Affairs.

Ireland, Expert Group on the Integration of the Income Tax and Social Welfare Systems (1996) *Integrating Tax and Social Welfare*, Dublin: Stationery Office.

Kennedy, K.A., Giblin, T. and McHugh, D. (1988) *The Economic Development of Ireland in the Twentieth Century*, London: Routledge.

Nolan, B. and Callan, T. (1994) *Poverty and Policy in Ireland*, Dublin: Gill and Macmillan.

Nolan, B. and Whelan, C.T. (1996) *Resources, Deprivation and Poverty*, Oxford: Clarendon Press.

Nolan, B., Whelan, C.T. and Williams, J. (1994) 'Spatial Aspects of Poverty and Disadvantage', in Nolan, B. and Callan, T. (eds) *Poverty and Policy in Ireland*, Dublin: Gill and Macmillan.

—— (1997) *Spatial Aspects of Poverty and Disadvantage: A Comparison of 1987 and 1994*, Dublin: Combat Poverty Agency.

O'Grada, C. (1994) *Ireland: A New Economic History 1780–1939*, Oxford: Clarendon Press.

Piachaud, D. (1987) 'Problems in the Definition and Measurement of Poverty', *Journal of Social Policy* 16 (2): 147–64.

Ringen, S. (1988) 'Direct and Indirect Measures of Poverty', *Journal of Social Policy* 17 (3): 351–66.

Rottman, D. (1994) 'Allocating Money Within Households: Better off Poorer?', in Nolan, B. and Callan, T. (eds) *Poverty and Policy in Ireland*, Dublin: Gill and Macmillan.

Sen, A. (1976) 'Poverty: An Ordinal Approach to Measurement', *Econometrica* 44 (2): 219–31.

Townsend, P. (1979) *Poverty in the United Kingdom*, Harmondsworth: Penguin.

World Bank (1996) *World Development Report 1996: Working in an Integrated World*, Oxford: Oxford University Press.

Chapter 6

Malta

Carmel Tabone

The Maltese Islands, consisting of Malta, Gozo and Comino, are collectively known as Malta. They are situated in the middle of the Mediterranean sea between Sicily and Northern Africa. The Islands cover an area of merely 316 square kilometres. The Maltese population, in 1993, amounted to 369,451, with a population density of 1,169 to the square kilometre (Malta, COS 1994).

MALTA: ITS HISTORY AND ECONOMY

History

Though small in area, Malta is very rich in history (Bowen-Jones *et al.*1962). This is reflected on the culture of the people. Its history which goes back to the Stone Age is characterised by the successive occupations of people of various cultures attracted by its central strategic position in the Mediterranean.

Neolithic temples and Megalithic remains show that the Islands were inhabited since the third millennium BC by people of a culture like that of the *stentinello* of eastern Sicily. Around 1450 BC the Phoenicians settled on the Islands and turned Malta into a trading station. The Carthaginians followed in around 550 BC. In the Second Punic War of 216 BC Rome took over and made Malta a *Municipium* of the Roman Empire.

The Arabs conquered Malta in around 870 AD, and remained on the Islands till 1090 when they were expelled by Count Roger of Normandy. Thus Malta was united to Sicily until 1530.

In 1530, Emperor Charles V of Spain ceded the Islands to the Knights of St John, who remained until 1798 when Napoleon took over Malta, during his expedition to Egypt. Very soon, however, the

Maltese turned against the French because of the latter's interference in religious and Church matters. They sought the help of the British, who took over in 1800, only two years after the French occupation. In 1918 with the Treaty of Paris, Malta became a British colony.

By the early decades of the twentieth century, the Maltese people wished to obtain their independence after a long history of foreign occupation. Their first attempt was the revolt of the so called *Sette Giugno* (seventh of June) of 1919, which was followed by the inauguration of the first Maltese Parliament and Constitution in 1921.

The aspirations of the Maltese for self-government reappeared when the Second World War was over. This resulted in the Constitution of 1947 which granted more authority in local affairs. The Maltese had to wait till 1964 to regain their independence, which was granted on 21 September of that year, when the Nationalist Party was in government.

On 13 December 1974, the Maltese Islands were declared a democratic republic, with a newly amended Constitution founded on work and respect of fundamental human rights and freedom of the individual.

The Labour Government sought to make up for the loss of revenue and employment from the withdrawal of British soldiers in 1979, mainly through the development of tourism and industry. The Labour Government sought also to extend commercial ties with North Africa and the Middle East, and Eastern Europe (Malta, Information Division 1982).

In 1987, the Nationalist Party won the general election. It sought to upgrade relations with Western countries. In 1990, Malta applied for membership within the European Union (EU), and since then the government made every possible effort to achieve this goal. For this reason the government thought of introducing VAT, in its pursuit to join the European union. VAT was introduced in 1995, while the government accepted an economic restructuring programme prescribed by Brussels as a condition of future membership in the (EIU 1994–5).

During 1993 and 1994, the political scene was dominated by the government's attempts to maintain a high employment rate and to sustain economic growth. The average unemployment rate during these years was around 4 per cent and the rate of GDP was about 5 per cent per annum in real terms. In 1993 inflation reached a maximum of 4.2 per cent, compared with the 1.6 per cent in 1992 (Brigulgio 1995).

The economy

One main characteristic of economic change impacting on the Maltese society has been the remarkably steady and sustained growth in the quality-of-life of the average Maltese family over the last decade. The Maltese economy averaged a real growth rate of 6 per cent between 1988 and 1991 and 4.5 per cent between 1992 and 1994, measured in terms of Gross National Product (GNP) (Malta, MEA 1994). The GNP per capita in 1993 was approximately US$8,000 (Briguglio 1995). The GNP is only an indicator of economic advancement. The GNP alone, however, may not be enough to indicate economic development. For a clearer idea of this development we need to consider other socio-economic measures that include quality-of-life indicators. In this regard one may consider the increase in television and radio licences, telephones and motor vehicles licences, education, electricity consumption, and social security. All these indicators registered a steady increase over these last ten years (Malta, MEA 1994).

In an international context Malta is usually classified as a developed country. In the United Nations Human Development Report, Malta is classified as a 'high human development country', with a Human Development Index (HDI) score of 0.886, ranking in the twenty-eighth place (UNDP 1996). Indeed, it can be claimed that the tastes and expectations of the Maltese compare well with those of developed countries. Many aspects of the standard of living and of the way of life of some Maltese are an exact copy of those found in high income economies. It seems to be the predicament of small states to have an obsession about measuring their life styles against those of foreign, especially ex-colonial, countries. The following words, uttered by the Prime Minister of tiny Montserrat (a British colony in the Caribbean) in the 1960s, may be applied to Malta as well: 'We live in a bicycle society with Cadillac tastes' (Thorndike 1985: 8).

THE CONCEPT OF RELATIVE POVERTY AND ITS MEASUREMENT

A definition of poverty

Poverty may be defined as economic deprivation. By this concise and rather simple definition any connotation in the concept of poverty which is not related to economic resources is excluded.

Social deprivation, for example, can easily be the cause of poverty, but it is not poverty. The two notions need to be distinguished. To consider any deprivation as poverty, including the physical deprivation (disability), would be a misnomer (Spanò 1992).

Such a distinction is necessary to safeguard the concept of poverty from dilution. By broadening the concept of poverty to include in it any non-economic deprivation there is the risk of shifting attention to other social problems, which are also real and call for concern, but discarding the economic deprivation. This is more likely to happen in the case of relative poverty. Absolute poverty is too evident to conceal. Not to give attention to relative poverty can be also ideologically motivated. Those having economic power and control, would not like to be constrained by any notion of a fairer economic distribution.

This broader sense of the term poverty, which includes every type of deprivation and almost any social problem, may have originated from the relation of the concept of poverty with that of human underdevelopment, where the latter has a much wider meaning than economic insufficiency. Human development aims at a general well-being of the person, which includes all aspects of human life, comprising the physical, economic, cultural, social and political dimensions (UNDP 1994). Human development is the promotion of all people and all that it is in people (*Popolorum Progressio*, 1967: n. 16).

Underdevelopment, therefore, is deficiency, or deprivation, in one or many of these aspects of human life, affecting the well being of the person, or persons. The equivocation of poverty and underdevelopment leads to the non-distinguishing of which aspect or aspects of human life is lacking and therefore causing underdevelopment. In this way, not every underdevelopment is poverty, only economic deprivation is. Underdevelopment is poverty when people lack economic resources in a relative or absolute sense, either because such resources are scarce, or because they happen to be unequally distributed.

Poverty in relative terms

A problem arises when one comes to determine deprivation in economic standards, especially in relative terms. When it concerns absolute standards, it is somewhat simpler to determine, as the lacking of basic needs is generally evident. But poverty has to be judged also relative to the productive capacity of society and to the standards between members of it (Lee and Newby 1987: 146; Abel-Smith and Townsend 1965; Rowntree 1941; Marshall 1994). It can be said that in relative terms the poor are those who live beneath the standard of living of a particular society. But again how is this standard determined?

One way of measuring relative poverty, in relation to the average standard of living, is to consider the quality of life of families. From the analysis of various indicators including income and expenditure, size and type of housing, as well as domestic and other familial commodities, an average standard of living can be obtained. This makes it possible to calculate which families are above it, and which are below that average quality-of-life.

This is the measure adopted by the author in a recent research project on the Maltese families (Tabone 1995), and the definition that will be adopted in this chapter. That study involved a simple random sampling survey of 559 heads of households, who were interviewed using a semi-structured questionnaire. Respondents were asked to evaluate the economic condition of their family so as to determine their expectations. It is both hard and risky to put families in conventional economic categories. But for the sake of analysis it is useful, as it serves to depict the actual economic condition of families, and determine the range and type of families which might be encountering financial difficulties, as well as the causes of such difficulties, when possible. This exercise gains significance when placed in the context of rapid economic growth, experienced in recent years, as formerly indicated.

This does not mean that such analysis is free from limitations, especially those often cited by critics of quantitative research. Indeed, to believe that a scientific and technical research design can, by itself, provide a completely valid and reliable picture of the focus of study may sound too pretentious. However, being fully aware of the danger of interpretation, research objectivity is still possible, while remaining respectful to the people under analysis and their vision.

QUALITY-OF-LIFE AND RELATIVE POVERTY

A picture of the quality-of-life and relative poverty of Maltese families can be derived from Tabone's 1995 survey (Tabone 1995), based on a number of basic indicators including income and expenditure, type and size of houses, as well as domestic and other familial commodities owned. It has been estimated, as resulting from the survey (Tabone 1995), that around 50 per cent of Maltese families were verging on the margin of relative poverty, while around 10 to 15 per cent other families lived in relative poverty.

Income and expenditure

Figure 6.1 shows that the average income of the Maltese family, as resulted from the analysis, is about Lm 260 monthly (mean: Lm 259.7). This amount is approximately equal to the social wage of a family with three children for 1993, which was estimated to be Lm 230 (*L-Orizzont* 30 September 1994), where the social wage is the minimum wage plus bonuses and allowances. For the purpose of this study, the average family is defined as a family with 2.76 children. The average income of a family of the same size, that is, parents and three children, as resulted from the survey, amounts to Lm 268 (mean: Lm 267.8). It appears, therefore, that the average family has generally speaking the average income. Around 60 per cent of families earn below the average income, while 40 per cent of families have an income which is above this average. There were 47.6 per cent who declared to be very much satisfied with the standard of living of their family. All others expressed some dissatisfaction about their families' standard of living. There were 10.8 per cent who stated that they were slightly or not at all satisfied with the standard of living of their family.

The issue of family expenditure was also assessed in the survey. For the purpose of the survey, expenditure has been defined as the amount of money the family deems necessary for ordinary purchases during a week. It can be taken to include what the family deems necessary for subsistence and other minor expenses, such as car fuel, clothing and leisure. For this reason, interviewees were asked how much their family needed *weekly* for living, and not how much it needed *monthly*, to avoid respondents including extraordinary expenses, and to make it easier for them to calculate ordinary ones. As defined, expenditure excludes house rent, mortgages, water and electricity bills, hire purchase instalments and other extraordinary expenses. However, information was also collected on the amount spent on water and electricity and telephone.

On the basis of the above definition of expenditure, it has been estimated that the average amount of money income deemed necessary by an average sized Maltese family for subsistence living was

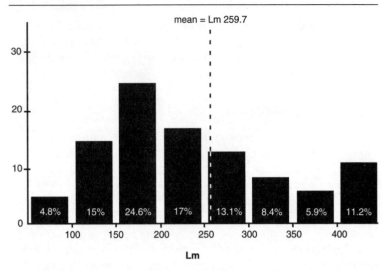

Figure 6.1 Percentage distribution of families' monthly income (in Maltese lira (Lm))

Lm 184 per month (mean: Lm 183.7), as shown in Figure 6.2. Around 55 per cent of the families spent less than the average expenditure for subsistence, while 45 per cent of families spent more.

It has been calculated that an average family with an average income was marginally above the relative poverty line. Some of these families seemed, at first glance, to save part of that income, but through further considerations it appeared that it would have been hard for them to do so. As stated, our definition of expenditure excluded water, electricity and telephone bills which on average amounted to Lm 16 per month in 1993, as calculated from the survey. Adding Lm 16 per month to this basic expenditure (Lm 184), the average family would have had a residual surplus of about Lm 60, given that the average income was Lm 260 per month. The difference between income and expenditure is being called residual rather than saving, as allowance has to be made here for the 'extraordinary' expenses excluded from the definition of expenditure given above. This may explain why 49.6 per cent of the respondents claimed that one wage was not enough, since with an average income it was hard to save. This matter, however, needs to be explored further.

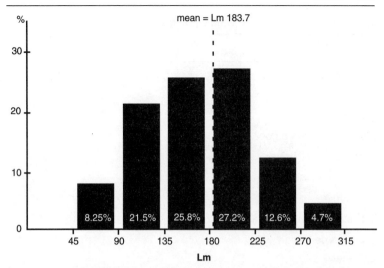

Figure 6.2 Percentage distribution of families' monthly expenditure for subsistence

Housing

Table 6.1 presents the results of the survey findings from Tabone's 1995 survey (regarding housing. It can be seen that the majority of the families seem to enjoy adequate housing in both size and quality, for 70.1 per cent live in one of the following type of houses: terraced house, maisonette, detached or semi-detached house. Around one quarter of families (26.8 per cent) live in a flat or one-storey dwelling on the ground floor.

As can be seen in Table 6.2, dwellings contained, in their great majority (over 90 per cent) the common necessary rooms namely: a kitchen, a sitting-room, two bedrooms and a bathroom. A similar majority (82.3 per cent) have a dining-room as well, while 56.4 per cent have more than two bedrooms. A significant minority (32.5 per cent) of the houses contained more than one bathroom. Only 10 per cent of the families declared having a second dwelling, typically a holiday resort.

Table 6.3 shows the availability of domestic appliances in Maltese households, according to the Tabone 1995 survey. Most homes were furnished with the necessary domestic appliances, including the telephone. There was a refrigerator, a washing machine, a gas or electric cooker, and a television in almost every

Table 6.1 Type of houses owned by Maltese families

Type of house	%
Terraced house	47.9
Flat	15.9
Maisonette	14.3
One-storey ground floor	10.9
Semi-detached house	5.2
Detached house	2.7
Farmhouse	0.7
Sub-standard housing (*kerreja*)	0.5
Special type (cellar)	0.2
No answer	1.7
	100.0

Source: Tabone 1995.

home. Three-quarters (76.4 per cent) of families had at least one car, while 24.5 per cent have more than one car. In 23.6 per cent of families there is no car. Only 4.5 per cent did not have a washing machine, which is significant in this day and age in terms of relative poverty or sub-standard quality-of-life conditions.

This relatively high standard of quality-of-life in the economy of

Table 6.2 Size of house owned by Maltese families (%)

Rooms	0	1	2	3	4+
Bedroom	–	7.6	36.0	47.8	8.6
Kitchen	0.4	98.5	1.1	–	–
Dining-room	17.7	79.2	3.1	–	–
Sitting-room	4.8	86.4	8.6	0.2	–
Bathroom	2.7	64.8	29.3	2.7	0.5
Garage	50.3	47.0	2.1	0.2	0.4

Source: Tabone 1995.

Table 6.3 Domestic appliances (%)

Appliances	0	1	2	3	4+
Cooker	0.7	94.4	4.7	–	0.2
Refrigerator	–	94.8	4.7	0.5	–
Deep freezer	58.9	38.6	2.3	0.2	–
Washing machine	4.5	85.3	9.1	0.9	0.2
Telephone	3.9	71.0	21.5	2.5	1.1
Television	0.4	66.0	28.3	4.3	1.1
Car	23.6	51.9	21.8	1.8	0.9
Air conditioner	94.6	4.5	0.2	0.7	–

Source: Tabone 1995

the families is reflected in the way they consider their standard of living (Broadbury 1989). Besides the 47.6 per cent who said that they were very much satisfied with the standard of living of their family, one may add that 41.1 per cent said they were moderately satisfied, revealing a degree of discontent. Overall, 80.3 per cent declared that they enjoy a higher standard of living than that of their family of origin.

INCIDENCE OF RELATIVE POVERTY

Nevertheless not all families seem to enjoy an average standard of living for a good quality-of-life, because 10.8 per cent stated that they are little or not at all pleased with their standard of living, and 14.5 per cent consider that their quality-of-life is not better than that of their family of origin. There were also 12.2 per cent of respondents stating that in their family one of the children had to seek employment to help the family to cope with its economic necessities. Families claiming an unsatisfactory quality-of-life standard need to be further examined to ascertain whether the sources of their dissatisfaction are purely economic (inadequate income) or because of their high expectations in comparison with their income earning capacity.

From further analysis, it transpired that families who considered that they were confronting economic difficulties, were in fact, in their majority, earning below the average level of income and thus in relative poverty. Those with the lowest levels of income form part of this category. These families considered that they were unable to cope on one wage alone. They were among those families having the highest number of presumably dependent children still living at home. The expenditure of families confronting economic difficulties was not above average, meaning that their economic expectations were not high. The average monthly expenditure of these families was Lm 164.

A marked difference was noticed between such families and those families, at the other end of the income spectrum, whose main breadwinners are employed in a high-level job as a result of their educational qualifications. The latter enjoyed better houses, with an expenditure higher than the average, declaring to be satisfied with their families' standard of living, although they too, considered that one wage is not enough. It is evident, that in this latter case one wage is not sufficient because the economic expectations tend to be very high. The average monthly expenditure of these families was Lm 210, well above average.

Sub-standard housing

In Tabone's 1995 survey (Tabone 1995), most of the families that confronted financial difficulties lived in sub-standard housing. It is difficult to identify exactly which houses were sub-standard, as some could be easily included under 'flat' or 'one-storey ground floor' for instance. Only 0.5 per cent considered that they live in a *kerreja* (Maltese for a sub-standard housing), while another 0.2 per cent lived in some type of cellar. On the basis of housing size data it can be concluded that around 8 per cent of the families had only one bedroom, 0.4 per cent did not even have a kitchen, let alone a dining-room, 2.7 per cent did not have a bathroom, and 4.8 per cent did not have a sitting-room. These dwellings are presumably small, and very likely to fall under the 'sub-standard' category. It is estimated that 10 per cent of families live in sub-standard housing. As already pointed out some families (4.5 per cent) do not even have a washing-machine. This is a significant figure, as the lack of such labour saving device, which has become a common household commodity, could not only be indicative of the quality-of-life these families experience, but also of their critical economic condition.

REASONS FOR THE EXTENT OF RELATIVE POVERTY

The reasons behind the conditions of families which considered they confronted financial difficulties were primarily economic, resulting from a wage that is inadequate to meet the expenditure needed, as appropriate to the size of their family with the average standard of living expectations. We can conclude that these families were relatively poor, as they were failing to achieve the average standard of living (Hutton 1991).

The amount of families living in relative poverty, as defined above, ranged from 10 per cent to 15 per cent of Maltese families, amounting to 11,500 of families in Malta. Loosely translated this would mean that around 23,000 adults and 31,500 children live in relative poverty in Malta, amounting to around 54,500 persons, 11.8 per cent of the population.

Families most affected by relative poverty

Families living in relative poverty were of four types. The largest group were those families headed by those in the younger age group (20–44 years of age), particularly those with low educational level and low occupational status, being unskilled labourers in the main. Generally speaking the occupation level is interdependent on the educational level (Hutton 1991). The second group are families with unemployed breadwinners who face financial difficulties and are not able to make ends meet. The third group are families comprising pensioners, widows and widowers, and the older age group (65 years of age and over). The fourth group are single-parent families, comprising unmarried parents and the separated.

SOCIAL WELFARE AND ANTI-POVERTY PROGRAMMES

Until 1990, social welfare in Malta was synonymous with social security. The development of social security on the Island could be traced back to the times of the Knights of St John who ruled the Island between 1530 and 1798. Under the Knights, the government provided social assistance to the poor in both cash and kind (mainly soup and bread). The poor included the disabled, retired soldiers and galley men, and/or their widows and orphans.

Under British rule, social security in Malta was regulated by three separate laws, namely: the Old Pension Act of 1948, the

National Insurance Act of 1956, and the National Assistance Act of 1956. This continued until 1987, when these acts were consolidated into a new Social Security Act. New programmes were added every now and than, especially after independence, to meet ever emerging new needs.

In 1974, two programmes were introduced: children's allowance and the handicapped pension. Children's allowances were paid under an amendment to the National Insurance Act, and were not subject to a means test. Initially, only the first three children under 16 years of age were eligible. But in 1977 coverage was extended to all children under 16.

The handicapped pension, as from 1994, was paid under the renamed disability pensions, including the Old Pension Act, which, as from 1957, already covered the blind. Now, both the physically and mentally disabled persons are covered, but a means test is applied.

In 1979, widows pensions were paid under the National Insurance Act. A national minimum pension was also introduced in 1979 to ensure that a contributory pension would not fall below a certain rate.

Maternity benefits were introduced in 1981. These were made available for everyone without means test or contribution conditions. Those who are already entitled to maternity leave on full pay were excluded.

The consolidated Social Security Act of 1987 was introduced to replace and establish afresh a social security system. Its purpose was: 'to consolidate with amendments existing provisions concerning the payment of social insurance benefits, benefits and allowances, social and medical assistance, non contributory pensions and the payment of social insurance, contribution by employees, employers, self-employed and the State' (The Social Security Act of 1987).

Notwithstanding this reform, new benefits continued to be introduced almost every year. In 1988 two new benefits were introduced: handicapped child allowance, which targeted handicapped children under the age of 16, and parental allowance, a means-tested benefit targeting families in financial difficulties.

Family bonus and short-term emergency assistance were two other benefits introduced in 1989. The former is an addition to the children's allowance benefits. The latter is a benefit in both cash and in-kind administered by the Director of Welfare to help destitute females who find temporary refuge in a home erected for this purpose.

In 1991, the widower's pension and orphans supplementary allowance were introduced. These non-contributory benefits targeted families that were dependent on the means of a deceased mother, or that had young children the care of whom required the widower to leave his employment.

In 1992, the carer's pension was introduced. This non-contributory pension compensates unmarried or widowed unemployed people who take care, on a regular basis, of an older and sick relative (De Gabriele 1994).

Free medical assistance including out-patient and in-patient services is a universal benefit. Polyclinics can be found in the main urban centres to provide medical care to the local population. Medication is distributed free of charge, as part of medical aid on a means-tested basis. The Health Services have co-operation agreements with other countries, particularly the United Kingdom. Serious cases are referred to hospitals in these countries.

With the publication of the white paper: *A Caring Society in A Changing World* in 1990 (Malta, MSP 1990), the government embarked on a national project to shift the Maltese society from a welfare state to a welfare society. The idea was to implement social policy on a more global basis, with wide-ranging measures that go beyond the limits of social security, while involving the greatest number of citizens possible in the promotion of a caring society. It meant a strategy intended to strengthen social justice in ways other than those purely financial.

The Ministry for Social Policy has been created for this purpose, which later became the Ministry for Social Development. Its objective is to co-ordinate the services provided by different departments (including health, labour, social security, welfare, the elderly and housing). This Ministry set up other structures within it to achieve its objective. These include: The Commission for the Advancement of Women, and the Department for Equal Status of Women, the National Commission for the Handicapped, and the Interdepartmental Commission Against Drug Abuse. Attention has been also given to the Voluntary Organisations (NGOs) in order to promote their valuable contribution to the achievement of social policy goals, as well as in building-up the welfare society philosophy.

The last structure to be set up within this Ministry of Social Development was the Social Welfare Development Programme (SWDP), which brings together different welfare units, including: the Community Development Unit, the Social Work Service on

Child Protection, the Social Work Service on Domestic Violence, the Development of Social Welfare Projects, the Social Work Service for Mental Health, the Family Therapy Services, and the Support Line Service (Malta, MSD 1994).

The Community Development Unit works with the people of socially deprived areas with the aim of developing human potential and improving and sustaining their quality-of-life by meeting their actual problems and instil in the community a development culture.

The Social Work Service in Child Protection deals with cases of suspected or reported neglected or abused children (including sexually abused).

The Social Work Service on Domestic Violence supports and empowers adult victims of domestic abuse, helps them to find shelter when needed and links them to other necessary services which they might also need. It works also with the perpetrators, helping them to control their violent behaviour.

The Development of Social Welfare Projects unit helps the Ministry for Social Development and other agencies to create and develop new services.

The Social Work Services in Relation to Mental Health is working on a reform project with social work regarding mental health.

The Family Therapy Services offer psychological help to families undergoing stress. It enables such families to have a better understanding of the nature of their problem and how to deal with it.

Finally, The Support Line Services is a telephone helpline providing accessible and confidential support and information to people in need (especially, with respect to child abuse, domestic violence and other problems).

These measures were highly instrumental in meeting and solving various social problems which might be related to poverty. However, poverty traps still exist, because the provisions of the welfare state are more on a blanket homogeneous basis, and therefore not always able to meet individual needs. In this way, some people fall out of the social security net and face financial difficulties. This contributes to the persistence of relative poverty in terms of economic deprivation, which needs direct attention to be reduced as much as possible.

REDUCING THE EXTENT OF RELATIVE POVERTY: FUTURE PROSPECTS AND STRATEGIES

Malta clearly enjoys quite an elaborate welfare state, with provisions updated regularly to meet ever emerging needs. This emerged to eradicate absolute poverty from the Islands. The isolated cases of absolute poverty that can be observed, are due to other social problems that often cause economic deprivation. One example is that of alcoholic breadwinners who spend all their income drinking thus depriving their family of their basic needs. Even in such cases, the spouse can still apply and receive assistance in cash, independent from the breadwinner. Nevertheless, relative poverty persists ranging from 10 per cent to 15 per cent of the families.

What could be done to eradicate relative poverty? Can the welfare state do this? Why does relative poverty persist, notwithstanding the existence of an elaborate welfare state? Tautologically, relative poverty persists for the simple reason that it is relative. It is not the aim of the welfare state to eradicate relative poverty, but to minimise its undesirable effects.

Relative poverty is a measure which compares and contrasts high income earners with low income earners, establishing a level of living that is below a particular benchmark or community accepted minimum standard that is related to both time and culture. The relatively poor in this study are those families whose income falls below the sum needed for average expenditure. One expects that the standard of living rises with the rise of the purchasing power which is dependent upon the income. In a free-market economy, there would be always those who fall below the average standard of living, whose purchasing power would not suffice for the expenditure needed to reach the community accepted minimum standard of living.

The welfare state was never aimed at ensuring that each and every citizen attains the average standard, in a continually rising standard of living of a particular society. A welfare state that aims to do this, is doomed to enter into a crisis, since in such a situation the state revenues would not suffice to meet the ever rising needs of its citizens. It should not be considered, however, that the aim of the welfare state is to ensure survival just above subsistence living (the absolute poverty line). The provisions of the welfare state needs to be in line with the actual standard of living of a particular society, but not so as to bring those who are wholly dependent upon social assistance onto the same standard of living level of those who are gainfully occupied. It can be agreed that this would lead to lack of initiative on the part of the citizen.

Work is the price that the people of Malta are paying for their satisfactorily high standard of living they are presently enjoying. The Maltese are hard workers, especially when this entails personal, individualistic or familial benefits. They are ready to undertake sacrifice in order to see their family enjoy a standard of living commensurate with a high quality-of-life. As they usually put it, no one would like to see one's family (standard of living implied) worse than that of others. Familism may contribute to economic advancement (Margavio and Mann 1989). Families have contributed to the economic advancement experienced in the last decade in their country. Had the welfare state sought to achieve equality in the standard of living for each and everyone, Maltese economic advancement would have been jeopardised. The welfare state provides a social safety net for those who cannot work. The welfare state is there also to help those who, notwithstanding their capacity for work, still remain below the average standard of living because their family dependants are too numerous and/or still young, or because the breadwinners are sick, disabled or dead.

Such arguments should never however imply that the persistence of relative poverty must be accepted fatalistically. Although relative poverty is from its very nature persistent, its extent can be limited. The state should aim to do this by reducing the gap between rich and poor. Towards this end the welfare state has to be maintained and updated regularly to meet ever changing community needs (Pierson 1991). Along with the welfare state, employment needs to be secured. Malta has actually enjoying a relatively low unemployment rate of 3.6 per cent over the last four years (Central Bank of Malta 1996), but this needs to be sustained.

The welfare state in Malta must in the future address some new community needs, especially in relation to those social categories that are most affected by relative poverty. The following are some suggestions as to what could be done in this regard.

The social wage, as defined previously, is to be revised regularly to match the economic needs necessary to maintain a socially acceptable minimum standard of living, and so reduce the risk of increasing the working poor. Social security measures need regular revision too so that they will be adequately assisting those families living in relative poverty. These measures entail further research and analysis to determine an official relative poverty line so that appropriate benefits rates can be set. It also calls for the need of a permanent monitoring network that would regularly revise the poverty line and social security measures related to it.

Measures are also needed to meet the needs of those living in poor or even sub-standard housing. Poor housing is one contemporary significant indicator of relative poverty in affluent Malta.

In addition, the delivery of community services, directed towards the family, need to be shifted from that based on blanket homogeneous provision, to one which is more specifically targeted. This should serve to promote a sensibility regarding the existence of different family types, with different needs. Needy families, and the type and amount of support they require, ought to be identified through social work assessment. Among the benefits which can be offered, training in social and home economics skills merit primary consideration. As a result, the process may also lead to the revision of the provisions of the social security schemes.

Another felt need is for area social workers who would be in a better position to identify the poor in particular geographical localities. This would help policy makers to take appropriate measures to respond adequately to the particular and personal needs of people.

CONCLUSION

Malta has gone a long way towards addressing the challenges of poverty. Absolute poverty has been virtually eradicated as a result of Malta's economic performance in recent decades and its willingness to invest in welfare state measures. Relative poverty, however, persists as a conspicuous symptom of inequality.

This chapter can be considered as an attempt to identify the characteristics of relative poverty, to quantify its incidence and to suggest measures to reduce its extent. Its basic argument is that it is only through the continuous improvement of the welfare state, that Malta will be able to keep relative poverty under control, minimising progressively its undesirable effects on Maltese society.

ACKNOWLEDGEMENTS

I am grateful to the students undertaking my course 'Sociology of the Family' at the University of Malta in 1995–6 for their useful help in the research necessary for this chapter.

REFERENCES

Abel-Smith, B. and Townsend, P. (1965) *The Poor and the Poorest*, London: Bell.

Bowen-Jones, H., Dewdney, J.C. and Fisher, W.B. (1962) *Malta Background for Development*, Newcastle-upon-Tyne: Durham College.

Briguglio, L. (1995) *The Economy of a Small Island State Malta 1960–1993, Mediterranean World*, Tokyo: The Mediterranean Studies Group, Hitotsubashi University.

Broadbury, B. (1989) 'Family Size Equivalence Scales and Survey Evaluations of Income and Well-Being', *Journal of Social Policy* 18 (3): 283–308.

De Gabriele, C.L. (1994) 'Social Security in Malta' (unpublished), Malta: Department of Social Security.

Economist Intelligence Unit (EIU) (1994–5) *Country Profile: Malta, Cyprus*, London: The Economist.

Hutton, S. (1991) 'Measuring Living Standards using Existing National Data Sets', *Journal of Social Policy* 20 (2): 237–57.

Lee, D. and Newby, H. (1987) *The Problem of Sociology*, London: Hutchinson University Library.

Malta, Central Bank of Malta (1996) *Quarterly Review* 29 (1).

Malta, Central Office of Statistics (COS) (1994) *Demographic Review of The Maltese Islands*, Malta: Government Press.

Malta, Information Division (1982) *Malta Handbook*, Malta: Government Press.

Malta, Ministry for Economic Affairs (MEA) (1994) *Economic Survey, January-September 1994*, Malta: Government Press.

Malta, Ministry for Social Policy (MSP) (1990) *A Caring Society in a Changing World: Proposals for a Social Welfare Strategy for the Nineties and Beyond*, Malta: Ministry for Social Policy.

Malta, Ministry for Social Development (MSD) (1994) 'Social Welfare Reform', 4 vols (unpublished report), Malta: Ministry for Social Development.

Margavio, A.V. and Mann, S.A. (1989) 'Modernization and the Family: A Theoretical Analysis', *Sociological Perspectives* 32 (1): 109–27.

Marshall, G. (ed.) (1994) *The Concise Oxford Dictionary of Sociology*, Oxford and New York: Oxford University Press.

Pierson, C. (1991) *Beyond the Welfare State*, Philadelphia, PA: The Pennsylvania State University Press.

Popolorum Progressio (1967) Encyclical Letter of His Holiness Pope Paul VI on the Promotion of the Development of Peoples, 26 March 1967, AAS 59, pp. 257–99.

Rowntree, B. S. (1941) *Poverty and Progress*, London: Longmans.

Spanò, A. (1992) 'La Povertànel Meridione: Caratteristiche del Problema, Aspettti Metodologici e Strumenti di Lotta', *Inchiesta* 22 (96): 59–71.

Tabone, C. (1995) *Maltese Families in Transition: A Sociological Investigation*, Malta: Ministry for Social Development.

Thorndike, T. (1985) *Grenada: Politics, Economy and Society*, London: Francis Pinter.

United Nations Development Program (UNDP) (1994) *Human Development Report 1994*, Oxford and New York: Oxford University Press.

—— (1996) *Human Development Report 1996*, Oxford and New York: Oxford University Press.

Chapter 7

Netherlands

*Henk-Jan Dirven, Didier Fouarge
and Ruud Muffels*[†]

The Netherlands is a rather small country (some 41,000 square kilometres of land) and had little less than 15.5 million inhabitants in 1995, which means it has a high population density of 452 people per square kilometre (Netherlands, Statistics Netherlands 1996a).

THE PROFILE OF THE NETHERLANDS

Demography

Although the Dutch population can be considered to be rather young when compared to other European countries, there is growing concern about the consequences of the ageing process of the Dutch population in the near future. While the percentage of young people (aged 19 or less) decreased between 1985 and 1995 from 28.3 to 24.4, the percentage of elderly (aged 65 or more) increased slightly from 12.0 to 13.2 (Netherlands, Statistics Netherlands 1992, 1996a). In the next 20 to 40 years, the percentage of elderly of 65 years and older will increase to 17 in 2015 and to almost one-quarter of the population in 2035 (Netherlands, Statistics Netherlands 1996b). In 1994, 31.1 per cent of all households were one-person households and 0.5 per cent were lone parent families (Netherlands, Statistics Netherlands 1996a).

[†] The research underlying this chapter was carried out while the first author was at Tilburg University. The views expressed are those of the authors and do not necessarily reflect the views or policies of Statistics Netherlands.

Socio-economic conditions

In the 1990s, the Netherlands has build up a remarkable economic record. Apart from a moderate annual inflation rate of 2.0 per cent over the period 1985–94, the Dutch Gross Domestic Product (GDP) per head is higher than the European Community (EC) average (see Table 7.1). Moreover, in the Netherlands, the real annual GDP growth rate per head was 1.8 per cent during the 1985–93 period whereas it was 1.6 per cent in the EC. Having an economic growth between 2.5 and 3 per cent in 1996 and an inflation rate just below 2 per cent, the Netherlands stands out economically among the other member states of the EC. Such achievements could be pursued due to a relatively high labour productivity and despite the rather low labour participation rate (see Table 7.1). Although female labour force participation showed a sizeable increase between 1985 and 1994, it still remains at a rather low level. While Dutch unemployment rates are rather low compared to the EC average, the Netherlands is confronted with a high rate of long-term unemployment. The increase in the working population between 1985 and 1991 and the falling unemployment rate reflect the favourable economic conditions. However, one should keep in mind that the increase in the working population went hand in hand with an increase in the number of part-time jobs and flexible labour contracts. In 1994, 36.4 per cent of the workers were employed in a part-time job (37.4 per cent in 1995) while 10.9 per cent were employed on a temporary basis (OECD 1996).

Social protection

The Dutch welfare state is often pictured as having one of the most equitable, generous and comprehensive social protection systems. Income policies have produced a high degree of income equality. Social protection expenditure as a percentage of GDP is higher in the Netherlands than in any other EC country. Social protection expenditure per head is also quite sizeable (one-quarter higher than the EC average in 1993). However, annual growth between 1985 and 1993 averaged 2.3 per cent, a lower growth rate than the EC average of 3.6 per cent. The share of sickness and invalidity benefits in total social protection benefits was equal to 43.1 per cent in 1985 and it increased to 44.6 per cent in 1993. The share of old age and survivors pensions in total social expenditure is also quite

Table 7.1 Summary statistics for the Dutch economy and the European Community in 1985, 1991 and 1993–4

	The Netherlands			European Community[a]		
	1985	1991	1993	1985	1991	1993
GDP/head[b, 1] (UK£)	6,887	7,873	7,884	6,147	6,966	6,957
Labour force participation[2, 3, 4] (%)	49.7	56.9	58.9[c]	54.3[d]	54.6	55.0[c]
males (%)	65.7	70.0	70.4[c]	69.0[d]	67.5	66.6[c]
females (%)	34.1	44.3	47.7[c]	40.9[d]	42.6	44.2[c]
Unemployment rate[2, 3, 4] (%)	10.5	7.3	7.2[c]	9.5	8.5	11.4[c]
Social protection expenditure in % of GDP[5]	31.7	32.4	33.6	26.0	26.0	27.8
Social expenditure per head[b, 5] (UK£)	2,181	2,521	2,585	1,604	1,930	2,067

Source:
1 Eurostat (1995a)
2 Eurostat (1987)
3 Eurostat (1993)
4 Eurostat (1996)
5 Eurostat (1995b).

Notes:

a The EU includes Belgium, Denmark, France, Germany, Greece, Ireland, Italy, Luxembourg, the Netherlands, Portugal, Spain and the United Kingdom.

b The data on GDP and social security expenditure presented in this table are expressed in UK pounds sterling at constant 1985 prices.

c The data are for 1994

d Spain and Portugal not included

substantial (32.7 per cent in 1985 and 37.1 per cent in 1993). The share of unemployment protection expenditure decreased from 11.6 per cent in 1985 to 9.2 per cent in 1993, mainly as a result of the falling unemployment rate.

The societal and political organisation of the welfare state in the Netherlands has typical corporatistic features through its traditional pillar-structure. Christians, Protestants, Socialists and Liberals were in separate organisations and tried to influence the form and content of the welfare state through their representatives in the decisive social and political bodies. This has characterised the Dutch welfare state over the period from the Second World War up to the early 1980s. The social protection system in the Netherlands is a mixed system which embodies elements of the Bismarckian and the Beveridgian welfare state models. According to others, the Dutch system combines elements of Esping-Andersen's typology of social democratic, corporatist and the liberal models (Engbersen *et al.* 1993). The first employee insurance scheme, which was introduced in 1901, covered the risk of accidents at work. Thereafter, disability, sickness and unemployment insurance were introduced. These employee insurance schemes were of the Bismarckian type: they were organised through the state, they were categorical since they covered the working population (*werknemersverzekeringen*) only and they were based on compulsory contributions levied on the wage bill. The old age and survivors pensions, as well as the family benefit scheme, were of the Beveridgian type (flat-rate pensions). They were universal since they covered the whole adult population, they were financed through contributions to be paid by the whole population (*volksverzekeringen*) or through general taxation. Still, most of the social protection benefits are contributory and insurance based. General assistance benefits on the other hand are financed through general taxation. The General Assistance Act was introduced in 1965 and was inspired by liberal views on the role of the state as provider of last resort. Assistance benefits are uniform, at a minimum level and means-tested by taking income from other sources (that is, both insurance benefits and earnings) within the household as well as savings and assets into account. Liberal ideas also have had a clear impact on the unemployment and health insurance schemes.

Political environment

The political context of the Netherlands is characterised by a long tradition of coalition governments. Three coalitions under the direction of the Christian Democrat Prime Minister Ruud Lubbers have dominated the political context: Lubbers I government (centre-right coalition 1982–6), Lubbers II government (centre-right coalition 1986–9) and Lubbers III government (centre-left coalition 1989–94). The main policy issues of the Lubbers I government were the reduction of public spending and the budget deficit, economic recovery and the restoration of employment (Roebroek 1993). The reform of the social protection system was also part of the political agenda, particularly with respect to health care, health insurance, family care and the level of the benefits (Roebroek 1993). The retrenchment policies to cut down government spending and reduce the budget deficit was continued during Lubbers II government. This government carried out a far reaching reform of the social protection system, particularly with respect to disability and unemployment benefits (lowering of benefits and reducing their duration). The Lubbers III government tried to reduce the budget deficit by limiting public spending through a further reform of the employee disability scheme, and through adjustments in health care programmes. With respect to disability, the policies of Lubbers II government were particularly aimed at reducing the number of recipients by reducing the flow out of employment, by a penalty on quits and lay-offs of disabled people, and by providing financial incentives to hire disabled peopled. Lubbers III government also aimed to privatise the disability scheme by reducing the legal protection against disability risks, by differentiating premiums according to the distribution of disability risks across firms and business sectors, and by giving greater responsibility to employers and employees within the framework of collective labour agreements (*Collectieve Arbeidsovereenkomst*) to determine the appropriate coverage of disability risks.

POVERTY IN THE NETHERLANDS

The definition of poverty

In the Netherlands, both in the political and the scientific debate, there is no consensus about the definition of poverty and its relationship with other concepts, such as social exclusion, deprivation, relative deprivation, marginalisation, disadvantage and social disadvantage. This chapter draws upon a conceptual framework which distinguishes between the concepts of income poverty, relative deprivation, impoverishment and social exclusion (Berghman 1995). The framework is, first of all, based on the distinction between income poverty (that is, lack of income) and relative deprivation (that is, inadequate living conditions). Second, it differentiates between static and dynamic perspectives.

According to Ringen (1988), poverty can be defined and measured in two ways: directly and indirectly (related distinctions were made by Sen (1979) between the direct method and the income method and by Atkinson (1987) between the right to a minimum level of resources and the attainment of a minimum standard of living). A direct definition of poverty focuses on relative deprivation; poverty is viewed as having unfavourable living conditions (broadly defined in terms of food, clothing, accommodation, social participation, education, work and social contacts). Such a definition is termed direct because it focuses on the actual spending patterns and living conditions of individuals. An indirect definition of poverty is aimed at measuring poverty using an indirect yardstick for consumption and living conditions, such as disposable income.

Under the indirect definition of poverty – the subsistence definition – people are poor if they do not have at their disposal the minimum amount of resources considered necessary to achieve a certain minimum living standard. This minimum amount of resources is called the subsistence minimum or the income poverty line.

The direct definition of poverty – the deprivation definition – states that individuals are poor if their living conditions lag behind what is considered to be just sufficient in the society in which one lives. The direct definition is therefore based on the person's actual living conditions, whereas the indirect definition is based on income as one of the determinants of these conditions. Research for the Netherlands (Dirven and Berghman 1991; Muffels 1993) indicates that income poverty is not the sole determinant of relative deprivation; other economic and social and cultural resources, appear to have an independent impact as well.

Poverty definitions may thus be classified into indirect (definitions of income poverty) and direct (definitions of relative deprivation). While the former are based on a uni-dimensional perspective on poverty in terms of a lack of income, the latter usually take a multi-dimensional perspective in terms of people's actual living conditions. Both concepts are used in a static sense, referring to the situation of individuals at a specific point in time. According to Berghman (1995), a distinction should be made between concepts referring to situations and concepts referring to processes. Table 7.2 displays the four possible combinations of direct and indirect definitions of poverty on the one hand, and static and dynamic definitions on the other hand. The concept of impoverishment may be used to denote the processes leading to income poverty, while the concept of social exclusion can be used to refer to processes bringing about a situation of relative deprivation.

As processes, impoverishment and social exclusion refer to chains of events causing people's income and living conditions to deteriorate to the extent that a situation of income poverty or relative deprivation occurs. Both processes may be triggered by changes in people's employment status as well as changes in family composition and may be affected by structural features of the labour market and the system of social protection (for example, (minimum) wage regulations, implicit tax rates and benefit levels). Moreover, due to stigmatisation, discouragement effects or moral hazard behaviour, previous situations of income poverty and relative deprivation may contribute to the processes of impoverishment and social exclusion. In this chapter, an analysis is carried out of the incidence of income poverty and relative deprivation and its evolution in the period under investigation. We will also draw attention to the flows into and out of poverty and the distinction between persistent and temporary poverty which is extremely important from a policy point of view. For further information on the processes of impoverishment and social exclusion the reader is referred to other publica-

Table 7.2 The conceptualisation of social exclusion and poverty

	Process	*Situation*
Indirect definition	Impoverishment	Income poverty (insecurity of subsistence)
Direct definition	Social exclusion	Relative deprivation (social disadvantage)

Source: Berghman 1995.

tions (Muffels 1993; Dirven and Fouarge 1995, 1996; Fouarge and Dirven 1995).

The incidence of poverty

This section presents results on the incidence of poverty in the Netherlands. The focus is, therefore, on income poverty and relative deprivation. The methods used to measure income poverty and relative deprivation are discussed briefly. The results are based on the Dutch Socio-Economic Panel Survey (Lemmens 1991), which is carried out by Statistics Netherlands and covers about 5,000 households. These households are interviewed annually (bi-annually until 1989). The most recent and comprehensive available data relates to the 1985–91 period, which is analysed below. A summary of more recent income poverty data for the period 1985–95, is drawn from the recently available waves of the Dutch Socio-Economic Panel Survey (SEP). Unfortunately, due to major changes in the questionnaire of the SEP, it appeared to be impossible to update the results on the incidence and persistence of relative deprivation.

Income poverty lines

In this section, two income poverty lines are used to determine income poverty during the period 1985 and 1991: the National Social Minimum Income (NSMI) and the Subjective Poverty Line (SPL). These poverty lines have in common that they are not imposed by the researcher, but have been drawn by politicians and the population, respectively. The National Social Minimum Income is based on political consensus (or, at least, on a majority view) as regards the minimum subsistence level. The Subjective Poverty Line is rooted in the everyday experiences of individuals trying to make ends meet (van den Bosch 1994).

Although no official income poverty line exists in the Netherlands, the amounts given in the General Assistance Act can be taken as the level of income which is considered by the authorities as the minimum income level necessary to live in subsistence. The amounts are dependent on the composition of the recipient's household, his or her age, and whether or not he or she shares a home. In determining the National Social Minimum Income level, not only general assistance benefits but also holiday allowances, incidental benefits, family allowances and student grants are included in the calculations.

The Subjective Poverty Line (Goedhart *et al.* 1977) is based on the judgements of heads of households about the minimum income required for their household. Although the adjective 'subjective' may perhaps suggest otherwise, this poverty line is not a purely subjective one. It refers to the fact that calculating the level of the Subjective Poverty Line is based on the subjective judgements of heads of households, taking as the point of departure their answers to the so-called minimum income question: 'What net income do you consider to be the absolute minimum for your household in your circumstances? In other words: if you had any less, you would not be in a position to make ends meet.' From these judgements an average or inter-subjective judgement is derived.

The answer to the minimum income question appears to be related to the composition of the household, the actual household income and the average income of the household's reference group, defined here as people with the same age and educational level. It can be shown that a level of income exists such that for all incomes below this level the income of the household is lower than the minimum income, whereas for all incomes above this level the income of the household is higher than the minimum income. This level of income is called the Subjective Poverty Line; it is the point at which households can just make ends meet.

In general, the level of the Subjective Poverty Line is higher than the level of the National Social Minimum Income. Apparently, the opinions of politicians and the population differ with respect to the level of the subsistence minimum. In order to determine income poverty, the level of the National Social Minimum Income and the Subjective Poverty Line is compared with the annual disposable income of the household. The latter is determined on the basis of a list of twenty-seven income components and includes the incomes of all household members. A person is considered to be in a situation of income poverty if the annual disposable income of the household to which he or she belongs, is lower than the National Social Minimum Income or the Subjective Poverty Line.

The incidence of income poverty: 1985–91

Table 7.3 presents results on the evolution of income poverty in the Netherlands between 1985 and 1991. For that purpose, the panel data are analysed as if they represent a series of repeated cross-sections. This enables trend analyses to be carried out, which gives insight into changes in the incidence of poverty and its distribution across population subgroups.

As far as the incidence of income poverty is concerned, the data indicate that, in 1990, about seven per cent of the Dutch population lived below the National Social Minimum Income, while about 11 per cent lived below the Subjective Poverty Line. Moreover, the situation has become somewhat worse between 1985 and 1990. The proportion of poor people was higher in 1990, irrespective of the income poverty line.

Engbersen, Vrooman and Snel (1996) present more recent figures on the incidence of income poverty. These show a slight decrease in the proportion of households below the social minimum during the first half of the 1990s, while the average amount of money needed to lift these households up to the level of the social minimum (the poverty gap) appears to have increased. However, due to the use of other definitions and data sources, their figures are not comparable to those presented in Table 7.3.

Poverty persistence: 1985–91

The richness of the panel data allows us to investigate the flows into and out of poverty and to assess whether poverty is temporary or persistent for particular groups in society. Following Bane and Ellwood (1986), a poverty spell approach is adopted here where a poverty spell is assumed to start after an individual being out of poverty in a particular year moved into poverty in the year after. The measure is based on the standard life-table approach. Income mobility is then defined in terms of the exit rate out of poverty,

Table 7.3 The evolution of income poverty, 1985–90: percentage of persons below the National Social Minimum Income (NSMI) and the Subjective Poverty Line (SPL)

	1985	1986	1987	1988	1989	1990
NSMI	6.4	6.4	6.7	6.1	5.4	6.7
SPL	9.6	11.7	12.8	12.4	9.7	11.1

Source: Muffels, Dirven and Fouarge 1995.

conditional on experiencing a poverty spell during specific time periods. In this approach, the survival rate after n years of poverty (that is, the proportion of people that did not escape) provides an estimate for the persistence of poverty.

The results of Table 7.4 show that there is a high income mobility in the Netherlands. Most poverty spells tend to end within two years. Notice that the mobility is much higher according to the National Social Minimum Income than according to the Subjective Poverty Line. This may be attributed to the lagged response of income evaluations to actual changes in income. Information for the Netherlands from other work (Duncan *et al*. 1993) show that beginnings and endings of poverty spells are to a large extent related to labour market events (losing or getting work, reduced or increased working hours) and household formation events (divorce or separation, (re)marriage). There is also evidence that in the period 1985 to 1991 the poverty status of groups with high annual risks on poverty, such as lone mothers, widows, long-term unemployed and disabled people, became worse through increasing persistent poverty (Muffels *et al*. 1995). Further analyses show that this is most likely attributable to falling escape rates out of poverty. The most recent figures published by Statistics Netherlands (1996c) on the numbers of households on a persistent low income indicate that this situation has continued during the first half of the 1990s. Periods of economic upswing obviously provide no guarantee for solving the issue of poverty. On the contrary, it appears that increasing labour market opportunities are preserved for a selective

Table 7.4 Long-term poverty according to the 'poverty spells' indicator and two poverty lines: the National Social Minimum Income (NSMI) and the Subjective Poverty Line (SPL); survival rate (%): 1985–90

Poverty spells (survival rate after n-years)	1	2	3	4
NSMI				
Total population	28.7	13.9	2.5	0.0
SPL				
Total population	56.3	39.2	26.1	23.4

Source: Muffels, Dirven and Fouarge 1995.

group of people. This means that for poor people with a very low chance of acquiring a regular job, the likelihood of moving out of poverty will not rise and poverty will become more persistent.

The incidence of income poverty: 1985–95

Table 7.5 presents results on the evolution of income poverty in the Netherlands between 1985 and 1995. Since the data were released in June 1997, it was not feasible to derive the National Social Minimum Income level and the Subjective Poverty Line for this statistical update. Instead, two other indicators of income poverty were used.

First, the incidence of income poverty was determined by taking all individuals living in households below 50 per cent of median standardised household income. This criterion is a common measure of income poverty used by the European Commission's statistical office (Eurostat) and independent researchers throughout the European Union. Second, figures are presented on the percentage of persons living in households having difficulties living within their household income. These figures are based on the answers to an income evaluation question phrased as follows: 'How did you get along with your household income in the previous twelve months?' If the answer was 'very difficultly' or 'difficultly', the household was considered to have difficulties to get along.

The poverty rates according to the 50 per cent of the median criterion indicate that, throughout the 1985–95 period, income poverty remained within the range of about 8 to 10 per cent of the Dutch population. The percentage of individuals living in households having difficulties to get along, on the other hand, fell dramatically in the second half of the eighties. This was followed by a slight increase during the first half of the 1990s. In 1995, about 11 per cent of the Dutch population lived in a household having difficulties to get along.

Poverty persistence: 1985–95

Using the indicators presented above, it is now possible to study the persistence of income poverty during the 1985–95 period. In Table 7.6, the persistence of poverty is analysed using the life-table approach. It displays the proportion of all poverty spells which started during the observation period (including multiple spells if

Table 7.5 The evolution of income poverty, 1985–95: percentage of persons below 50% of median standardised household income and living in households having difficulties getting along

	Below 50% of median standardised household income*	Having median difficulties getting along
1985	8.5	18.4
1986	8.2	15.8
1987	8.3	13.8
1988	8.6	11.6
1989	8.6	10.2
1990	10.0	–
1991	8.6	9.0
1992	8.8	9.3
1993	9.5	10.0
1994	9.4	12.3
1995	–	11.4

Note:

*As of 1990, the measurement of income was changed from current monthly income (in October) to income in the previous year. The figures have been adjusted in order to be comparable across the whole period.

an individual became poor more than once) and continuing after one year, after two years, and so forth. Survival rates are indicative of poverty persistence.

The results show that most poverty spells end after one year. Income poverty thus appears to be a short-term situation for most people. There is, however, a remarkable difference between the two poverty definitions. The survival rates below 50 per cent of median standardised household income decrease more slowly with duration than those in a situation where individuals are living in households which have difficulties to get along. While 21 per cent of the former spells continue after five years, this is true only for 7 per cent

Table 7.6 Long-term poverty according to the poverty spells indicator using below 50% of median standardised household income (1985–94) and having difficulties getting along (1985–95)

Poverty spells
(cumulative survival rate after n-years)

	1	2	3	4	5*
Below 50% of the median	44.2	32.7	26.7	20.9	20.9
Difficulties to get along	41.2	22.6	13.9	9.1	6.8

Note:

* Due to the low number of observations, the cumulative survival rates for six years or more are not included in the table.

of the latter spells. Apparently, low income situations are more persistent than feelings of income deprivation.

Relative deprivation: 1985–91

While income poverty lines may be used to describe the income situation of households, relative deprivation indices are employed to study situations of multiple disadvantage. Following the works of Townsend (1979), Mack and Lansley (1985) and Desai and Shah (1988) on the definition and measurement of relative deprivation, Muffels (1993) developed a Subjective Deprivation Poverty Line. It is based on the majority view of the Dutch population about the living conditions which are considered sufficient for a given type of household.

The derivation of the Subjective Deprivation Poverty Line involves two main steps. First, the extent of relative deprivation of a household is determined using a so-called subjective deprivation scale. This scale consists of a list of items reflecting people's living conditions. The extent of deprivation is calculated as a weighted sum of the score on each item that the individual considers as absolutely necessary to have. If he or she lacks an item, one is added to the deprivation score and if he or she possesses it, one is subtracted. However, while adding up and subtracting these items, weights were used reflecting the extent to which various items were possessed or lacked by the reference group of the household. The reference group was assumed to consist of households with heads having the same age and educational level.

The second step is to transform the subjective deprivation scale into a Subjective Deprivation Poverty Line. The transformation is based on the level of satisfaction expressed by the respondent with respect to his or her living conditions. This is measured by the so-called life resources evaluation question, which was asked directly after the list of items:

> If you consider the way in which your household lives at the moment, would you call your household poor, or in fact rich, or somewhere in between? You can answer by giving a score to your situation. A score of 1 means that you consider yourself to be very poor; a score of 10 means that you consider yourself to be very rich.

The level of the Subjective Deprivation Poverty Line is then assessed by assuming that there exists a level of deprivation below which people live in deprivation poverty and above which people do not live in deprivation poverty. The dividing line is found by assuming that, as with the school mark system in the Netherlands, a score of 5.5 reflects the dividing score between 'satisfactory' and 'unsatisfactory' which can therefore operate as the threshold level with respect to the evaluation of one's living conditions. The resulting Subjective Deprivation Poverty Line varies across household types, because the score on the answer to the life resources evaluation question is also influenced by reference group factors, age and marital status of the head of household, and indicators of financial stress. The latter is indicated by the head's opinion about the current financial situation of the household and by his/her financial expectations. The level of the poverty line can be taken to be the line which exists, according to the Dutch population, between a 'sufficient' and an 'insufficient' level of living conditions for a given type of household.

The incidence of relative deprivation: 1985–91

As Table 7.7 indicates, a substantial decrease in the incidence of relative deprivation was observed between 1985 and 1991 among both households and individuals. By the way, the proportion of relatively deprived households appears to be higher than the proportion of relatively deprived individuals. Apparently, relative deprivation is more common among smaller households. Moreover, the ratio of deprived to non-deprived households and individuals appeared to have decreased by about 10 per cent per year. Closer examination of the data showed that this was mainly caused by decreasing levels of the Subjective Deprivation Poverty Line, while the living conditions did not change on average. Apparently, the level of deprivation which is considered by the Dutch population to be the dividing line between satisfactory and unsatisfactory living conditions decreased between 1985 and 1991. Using different data and definitions, Engbersen *et al.* (1996) show that the average level of well-being increased slightly between 1991 and 1993. Since the bottom end benefited from this increase to the same extent as the rest of the population, it is argued that the incidence of relative deprivation remained at a stable level.

Deprivation-poverty persistence: 1985–91

To assess the persistence of deprivation status we had to impute the information for the years 1987 and 1989 for which we lacked information on deprivation. The predicted deprivation-poverty status can then be used to calculate the spell-based measure of income mobility and poverty persistence (Muffels and Dirven 1995). In Table 7.8 the results on the persistence of deprivation-poverty are given.

The results show that in general the stability of deprivation-poverty is higher than was found using the income-poverty lines and especially compared to the social minimum threshold. After

Table 7.7 The evolution of relative deprivation, 1985–91: percentage of households and percentage of persons below the Subjective Deprivation Poverty Line (SDL)

	1985	1986	1988	1991
SDL 5.5				
Households	14.0	13.2	11.6	9.0
Individuals	10.8	10.2	9.4	6.1

Source: Muffels, Dirven and Fouarge 1995.

Table 7.8 The persistence of subjective deprivation poverty according to the Subjective Deprivation Poverty Line (SDL); survival rate (%): 1985–91

Deprivation spells (survival rate after n-*years)*				
	1	*2*	*3*	*4*
Total population	47.8	27.2	27.2	27.2

Source: Muffels and Dirven 1995.

four years, about 30 per cent of the deprivation-poor had not managed to escape from poverty.

GROUPS MOST AFFECTED BY POVERTY

This section presents information on the distribution of poverty across population groups. The presentation is based on the social barometer of poverty in the Netherlands (Muffels *et al.* 1995), which provides an insight into the distribution of annual poverty rates across a large number of demographic and socio-economic background variables, such as sex, age, household type, educational level, and so forth.

Poverty profile in the early 1990s

The results presented in Table 7.9 refer to the most recent compa-rable data available on income poverty (1990) and relative depriva-tion (1991). Again, the National Social Minimum Income (NSMI) and the Subjective Poverty Line (SPL) were used to measure income poverty. Relative deprivation was operationalised by the Subjective Deprivation Poverty Line, using a level of 5.5 (between unsatisfac-tory and satisfactory) on the life resources evaluation question (SDL 5.5).

Underlying the social barometer of poverty are a number of demographic and socio-economic background variables. The selec-tion of variables is based on theory as well as on the observed impact from a multivariate analysis. Each of the variables included in the social barometer has a direct impact (net of the other variables) on the risk of being poor at a specific point in time. Of those, the following variables appeared to have the strongest effects: sex of the head of household, age of the head of household, marital status, position in the household, household type, socio-economic group of the head of household, socio-economic class of the head of household and the number of earners in the household. The distribution of poverty across population groups defined by those variables is discussed here.

Sex, age, marital status and household composition

As Table 7.9 indicates, income poverty is rather unevenly spread depending on whether the household has a *male* or a *female* head. The risk of being below the NSMI appears to be about three times as high for individuals living in a household with a female head compared to those living in a household with a male head. According to the subjective poverty lines (SPL and SDL), the differences are even larger. The distribution of poverty across *age groups* of the head of the household shows the lowest (16–24 years) and the highest (75 years and older) age groups to be consistently more prone to poverty.

Breaking down poverty by *marital status* of the head of household, it appears that individuals living in households with a divorced or widowed head have the highest risks of being poor. The risk of being relatively deprived is particularly high among those in households with a divorced head.

Table 7.9 also indicates that *single persons* generally have the highest risk of being poor. This is especially so according to the two subjective poverty lines (SPL and SDL) and to a lesser extent according to the NSMI. This conclusion partly reflects the results found for persons living in households with a female or divorced/widowed head and indicates that single divorced or widowed females have relatively high poverty risks.

One-person households as well as *single-parent households* have much higher risks of being poor than couples. Among couples, the presence of children does not increase the risk of being poor (rather the opposite). Non-family households (for example, students living in the same household) are less prone to poverty than other groups.

Table 7.9 Percentage of persons below the National Social Minimum Income (NSMI), the Subjective Poverty Line (SPL) and the Subjective Deprivation Poverty Line (SDL 5.5) by demographic and socio-economic background variables in the early 1990s

	NSMI (1990)	SPL (1990)	SDL 5.5* (1991)
Sex of the head of household			
male	5.1	6.9	3.1
female	16.3	36.0	23.1
Age of the head of household			
16–24	26.9	41.7	10.9
25–49	5.0	6.6	5.1
50–64	7.8	11.7	7.3
65–74	5.3	18.1	5.6
75+	9.6	27.5	10.8
Marital status of the head of household			
married	4.1	4.6	2.3
divorced	16.4	27.8	40.2
widow(er)	11.0	37.5	10.8
unmarried	14.4	25.8	7.6
Position in the household			
single	17.1	42.8	32.5
head of household	5.4	6.6	9.1
partner	4.5	5.4	7.9
child	4.9	5.3	7.4
other	2.2	6.5	6.5
Household type			
one-person household	17.1	42.8	16.7
non-family household	4.8	5.9	1.6
couple without children	5.2	7.3	2.9
couple with children	3.6	3.6	2.0
single-parent household	16.6	20.3	31.4
Socio-economic group of the head of household			
self-employed	9.4	11.8	4.8
public employee	1.7	2.4	1.9
private employee	3.4	4.4	2.0
unemployed	30.5	45.4	20.7
(early) retired	6.9	18.8	6.8
disabled	13.5	23.8	16.2
on general assistance	35.0	51.1	66.1
Socio-economic class of the head of household			
service class	1.8	2.5	0.9
routine non-manual	2.6	5.0	2.6
petit bourgeois	11.8	14.3	11.8
farmers	10.9	9.6	1.1
skilled workers	2.3	2.6	2.3
non-skilled workers	7.2	9.2	4.7
farm workers	13.9	17.1	0.0
Number of wage earners in the household			
0	16.6	32.4	16.1
1	5.1	7.5	4.3
2	2.8	2.5	1.7
3+	1.2	1.2	0.7

* The SDL was set at a level of deprivation which corresponds with a score of 5.5 on the life resources evaluation question. This score reflects the dividing line between satisfactory and unsatisfactory living conditions.

Source: Muffels, Dirven and Fouarage 1995

Socio-economic group, socio-economic class and number of earners

The distribution of poverty by *socio-economic group* of the head of household in Table 7.9 shows, first, that self-employed heads are more likely to be income poor than employees, although this differentiation applies much less to relative deprivation. This may be due to the differential evolution of self-employment income over time, which may be negative in one year (business losses), but fully compensated in the next (business profits). Secondly, people dependent on social protection benefits are more likely to be poor than people with a paid job. This holds except for the retired (including those on early retirement), who may be able to draw upon savings and/or whose subjective assessments of income may be more positive due to lower demands for income and lower income expectations. The poverty risks for employees would suggest that the *working poor* do not exist in the Netherlands. However, the increase of *atypical* and *flexible* jobs (that is, fixed-term, part-time and/or without fixed working hours), which have higher poverty risks than other workers, could make it an issue in the near future.

For persons living in households with an employed head, the social barometer includes information on poverty risks by *socio-economic class*. The classification into socio-economic classes used here was developed by Erikson, Goldthorpe and Portocarero (1979) and is based on information on the employment sector (manual, non-manual and agricultural work), skills, employment status (self-employed, employee) and supervision status (large owners/supervisors, small owners/supervisors, no supervision). As Table 7.9 indicates, farm workers, the petty bourgeoisie and farmers face high risks of being income poor, while relative deprivation stands out among the latter class only.

To conclude, this section briefly discusses the distribution of poverty in the early 1990s across households with different *numbers of wage earners*. Not surprisingly, poverty risks are highest among those without earnings. Among those with earnings, the risks decrease slightly with the number of earners in the household.

Poverty profile in the mid-1990s

Table 7.10 presents information on the groups most affected by income poverty in 1995. While the data refer to 1995, the 50 per cent of the median criterion was based on annual household income in 1994.

According to the 50 per cent of median standardised household income criterion, four groups appear to be most affected by income poverty in the mid-1990s, as in the early 1990s: households with a head aged 16–24, recipients of social assistance benefits, the unemployed and single-parent households. At least one in five of these groups are below the income poverty line. Moreover, the results indicate that most social assistance beneficiaries in the Netherlands have difficulties to get along with their income. In addition, single-parent households, the unemployed, divorced and female-headed households also have more difficulties than other groups. Poverty risks thus appear to be high for those on social assistance, the unemployed and single-parent households according to both criteria. While young heads of households are at risk of being below 50 per cent of median standardised household income, they do not display disproportionate difficulties getting along on their incomes. This may be explained from the transitory nature of their low income situation.

POLICY RESPONSES TO POVERTY

Up to the end of 1995, the Netherlands had no official anti-poverty programme, since it was believed that poverty hardly existed. There were programmes focusing on those with low incomes but the term poverty was expressly avoided. In the political debate on the social renewal policy (*Sociale Vernieuwingsbeleid*) at the beginning of the decade, emphasis was put on the concept of social disadvantage (*sociale achterstanden*), which refers to disadvantages in terms of income as well as living conditions. The concept of poverty was dealt with only occasionally in government reports on social policy. However, it was explicitly acknowledged that, despite the high level of the minimum guaranteed income, problems of social disadvantage were present in the Netherlands. Moreover, social disadvantage was characterised as a problem of non-participation in the labour market. The government argued that, while the Dutch system of social protection appears to be rather effective in alleviating financial distress, it is rather ineffective in increasing (full-time) labour market participation.

Various policy measures were proposed to create employment and lower the number of beneficiaries. These measures were aimed at increasing labour market participation and reducing

Table 7.10 Percentage of persons below 50% of median standardised household income and living in households having difficulties getting along by demographic and socio-economic background variables in 1995

	Below 50% of median standardised household income	Having difficulties getting along
Sex of the head of household		
male	8.8	8.6
female	13.4	29.6
Age of the head of household		
16–24	30.6	15.8
25–49	9.3	10.0
50–64	8.8	12.1
65–74	5.8	16.3
75+	4.8	12.7
Marital status of the head of household		
married	8.8	8.4
divorced	15.7	33.8
widow(er)	6.7	20.9
unmarried	10.4	10.8
Position in the household		
single	8.5	18.6
head of household	8.1	10.1
partner	8.0	8.1
child	12.2	12.1
other	28.1	15.4
Household type		
one-person household	8.5	18.6
non-family household	7.8	13.3
couple without children	4.5	6.8
couple with children	11.0	9.0
single-parent household	20.0	42.7
Socio-economic group of the head of household		
self-employed	11.2	9.7
public employee	1.8	5.2
private employee	3.4	6.7
unemployed	29.8	42.2
(early) retired	5.0	13.5
disabled	10.9	21.3
on general assistance	32.7	85.5
Socio-economic class of the head of household		
service class	1.4	4.0
routine non-manual	2.9	6.7
petit bourgeois	12.5	10.5
farmers	16.3	10.1
skilled workers	3.3	7.1
non-skilled workers	7.6	11.5
farm workers	3.0	11.9
Number of wage earners in the household		
0	17.4	23.5
1	12.7	10.7
2	2.2	5.1
3+	0.6	2.0

social disadvantage. Although the proposals were not explicitly framed in terms of poverty, they can be conceived as dealing with related problems. The aim of these policy measures is to intervene in the processes leading to relative deprivation and social disadvantage. Previously, we have referred to these as the process of social exclusion.

In its report on social policy, the present 'purple' coalition (consisting of Social-Democrats, Democrats and Liberals) under the direction of Social-Democrat Wim Kok proposed the following general policy framework (Netherlands, Second Chamber 1994). First of all, macroeconomic measures, such as wage restraint, tax decreases and shifts in the tax burden are considered necessary to increase employment. In that respect, tax decreases for low-paid jobs are regarded to be one of the main policy instruments. Second, in order to reduce problems associated with long-term unemployment, the government called on the social partners (that is, employer and employee organisations) to develop a common strategy to tackle persistent unemployment. In the meantime, employment programmes were set up by the Minister of Social Affairs and Employment, Horst Melkert, to create 40,000 additional jobs in the public sector (the so-called Melkert I jobs), followed by employment programmes for the creation of jobs in the private sector (Melkert II jobs) and the non-productive social sectors of the economy (Melkert III jobs). Third, a fundamental reform of the social protection system was proposed in order to increase incentives to participate in the labour market. The reformed system should meet the following new standards: its preventive function should be improved, its selectivity should be increased and recipients should be required to adopt a more active attitude towards the seeking of employment. More attention should be paid to private income protection schemes. And, last but not least, implementing bodies should be judged by their effectiveness.

On 24 November 1995, following the United Nations summit on poverty and social exclusion, a government report entitled 'The Other Side of the Netherlands' (*De andere kant van Nederland* (Netherlands, Second Chamber 1995) was presented to Parliament by the Minister of Social Affairs and Employment. The report is important because, for the first time, the government not only officially recognised the existence of poverty in the Netherlands but also accepted responsibility for tackling the problem. It thus ended a long period of denial and reluctance by government to substitute the term 'poverty' in official policy reports for the vaguer notion of 'social disadvantage'.

The current government explicitly aims at preventing and tackling problems of 'silent' or hidden poverty (*stille armoede*) and social exclusion. It claims that poverty in the Netherlands is a problem of people lacking social and economic opportunities. Poverty should therefore not be conceived *senso stricto*, that is, as referring to situations of hunger, physical hardship and starvation, such as is the case in Third World countries. Instead, poverty in the Netherlands is primarily a matter of 'silent' poverty hidden behind the curtains of prosperity. However, the government does not provide an explicit criterion to distinguish between overt and hidden poverty. In defining poverty, it adheres to the European Commission's definition of poverty:

> [T]he poor shall be taken to mean persons, families and groups of persons whose resources (material, cultural and social) are so limited as to exclude them from the minimum acceptable way of life in the Member State in which they live.
>
> (Hagenaars *et al*. 1994: 2)

It should be noted that this definition is relative: poverty is defined relative to the living standard of the member state where a person lives. Moreover, the definition is multi-dimensional: it combines various types of resources as well as people's actual living conditions.

Contrary to the definition of poverty, social exclusion is defined more vaguely in terms of a worsening of social living conditions, a restricted social network, the continuous use of strategies for survival and the lack of opportunities. Again, this is a multi-dimensional definition which combines various aspects of people's living conditions. Moreover, it suggests that social exclusion is a process and refers to changes over time.

The government's aim is to combat poverty and social exclusion using four policy strategies. The first strategy deals with employment creation. Employment policies pursue the creation of at least 350,000 jobs within the next four years (1996–9), especially at the lower end of the labour market. For those with very little opportunities to find a job (for example, women with young children, elderly persons, people with low educational attainments or severe social and psychological problems), the government promotes social participation by stimulating unpaid social activities and allowing benefit recipients to earn some additional income.

The second strategy aims to use the general assistance scheme as the safety net. This presumes that the government will protect the purchasing power of minimum benefits; that the effectiveness of the special assistance scheme will be assured; and that the income position of the elderly and families with children will be improved.

The third strategy requires that the amounts to be paid by low income households for fixed housing costs should be lowered and more households with financial problems should be guided and supported by local authorities. This includes measures to keep the costs of housing low, to reduce the municipal tax burden for low income households and to alleviate problematic debts.

The fourth strategy is to increase the take-up rate of entitlements to social protection by streamlining administrative procedures, by reducing and simplifying regulations, by improving the quality and quantity of programmatic information, and by harmonising income concepts.

EVALUATION OF ANTI-POVERTY PROGRAMMES

The proposals made by the government received broad support in parliament. Given the public recognition of the poverty problem, the desirability of anti-poverty programmes is hardly disputed (not even by the opposition, which mainly consists of Christian-Democrats). Naturally, it is too early yet to evaluate the specific measures introduced by the government. However, some evaluation was made of policies implemented by the previous centre-left Lubbers III government, which followed three main strategies to reduce social disadvantage. Employment creation programmes were perceived by the Lubbers III government as necessary but insufficient to solve the problem of social disadvantage. This strategy was supplemented by income policies, which required adjustments of the social protection system to increase work incentives. The third strategy tackled the problem of social disadvantage at the local level by means of the social renewal policy. A few examples of the previous government's policy to reduce the problem of social disadvantage are briefly discussed here.

The job pool and the youth employment guarantee schemes

Long-term unemployment (that is, being registered as unemployed for more than one year) amounted to 247,000 in 1995 (197,000 in 1990), which is 53.2 per cent (55.0 per cent in 1990) of all registered unemployed. To tackle long-term unemployment, the job pool scheme was introduced on 1 January 1991. It is aimed at persons being unemployed for more than 3 years. In a re-orientation talk, it is determined whether an indiviual applies for the job pool. At present, about 23,000 people participate in the scheme, the majority of whom are aged over 35 and who have been unemployed for more than five years. Municipalities are responsible for setting up or designating a job pool foundation which is able to hire unemployed people to work in additional jobs (that is, jobs which otherwise would not have been created) within public or non-profit organisations. Earnings are set at the level of the minimum wage.

Together with women, minorities and the low-educated, unemployed youngsters (that is, those below 25 years of age) are one of the target groups of the government's labour market policy. In 1995, 89,000 youngsters (85,000 in 1990) were officially registered as unemployed, which is 19.1 per cent (23.7 per cent in 1990) of all registered unemployed. In order to prevent long-term unemployment and to provide new opportunities for regular jobs, the youth employment guarantee scheme was introduced nationally on 1 January 1992. The scheme is a safety net provision offering a temporary job, at the minimum youth wage, after six months of unemployment. At present, it applies to school-leavers below 25 years of age (youngsters without any previous work experience) and to unemployed youngsters below 21 (youngsters who have had a previous job). In 1998, all school-leavers below 27 and unemployed youngsters below 21 will be covered. The scheme is carried out by a youth employment guarantee foundation and now provides about 23,000 additional jobs mostly in public and non-profit organisations. Every six months, participants of the programme are examined to evaluate their chances of entering the regular job market so as to assess whether they need additional training or work experience. If a job offer is rejected by the unemployed enrolled in the scheme, his or her unemployment benefit can be reduced.

The general assistance scheme

The general assistance scheme is the most important scheme for guaranteeing a minimum level of resources in the Netherlands. Moreover, it should be regarded as the foundation of the social protection system, since it renders a minimum income to those who can not draw benefits from other sources. The general assistance scheme provides (means-tested) financial assistance to every registered resident who can not adequately cover the necessary costs of living for his or her household. General assistance benefits are financed by the central government (90 per cent) and the municipalities (10 per cent). Municipalities have extensive discretionary powers to determine eligibility of benefits under the scheme. They also have the capacity to provide supplementary benefits meant to offset particular costs faced by the applicants. These special assistance benefits are financed entirely by the municipalities.

The social renewal policy

Crucial elements of the social renewal policy are the direct approach of the individual citizen, the breakdown of existing legal and financial barriers and the adoption of an integrated approach at the local level in order to increase social participation by means of employment. For this purpose, responsibility for allocating money from existing local budgets is transferred to local authorities and subsidised institutions to give them a greater capacity to adopt new approaches and methods to achieve social renewal. The role of the central government has been restricted in setting the general framework within which the local authorities have acquired greater discretionary power to take their own measures to combat social disadvantage. The social renewal policy did not involve any additional government funding but only an integration of existing budgets into one large fund by the central government. In practice, the social renewal policy hardly involved any new policy instruments. Many measures, such as wage and training subsidies, sheltered employment, social work and basic education. existed before social renewal was launched. Some municipalities also had an integral policy measure directed at area-related problems (bad housing, unemployment, low education): the problem-accumulation areas policy (*Probleem Cumulatie Gebiedenbeleid*). What was really new about the social renewal policy was, most of all, its administrative nature (Oeij 1993).

Evaluation

Some evaluation studies have been conducted on programmes aiming to reduce social disadvantage. Their efficiency and efficacy was considered to be disappointing (Serail and Ter Huurne 1995). In most instances, the programmes did not reach the most disadvantaged among the target groups, while those who did participate probably would have improved their situation anyway. The impact of these programmes on the increase of labour market opportunities of the participants was estimated to be modest. Also, doubts were raised about the extent to which additional jobs were created that did not compete with regular jobs.

However, even if labour market policies fail to reduce aggregate levels of unemployment, it could be argued that they contribute to increasing mobility into and out of unemployment. And, of course, there may be good arguments to prefer an open society where the burden of unemployment is shared between many people for a short period of time to a society with an underclass of long-term unemployed people. Nevertheless, the available evidence on the mobility of the unemployed (Ultee *et al.* 1992) does not render much support for the proposition that these programmes enhance labour market mobility.

Evaluations of the Dutch general assistance system show that its efficacy in terms of reducing the poverty rate and poverty gap is high (Deleeck *et al.* 1992; Commission of the European Communities 1994). While, in 1986, the Netherlands had a poverty rate of 39.8 per cent before social protection benefits were received (using the 50 per cent of average disposable household income poverty line), it succeeded in reducing this figure by 82 per cent to 7.2 per cent after the receipt of social protection benefits. Moreover, the poverty gap was reduced by 90.9 per cent. However, like in the other member states, the system appears to be rather target inefficient. Almost half of the aggregate cash transfers goes to households that were at, or above, the National Social Minimum Income level without social protection transfers, or to households in excess to what they strictly need to stay above that level. Finally, research on the take-up of benefits (van Oorschot 1991) indicates that serious problems exist with respect to granting the least privileged their legal rights.

Evaluation studies of the Dutch social renewal policy (Oeij 1993; van der Wouden *et al.* 1994), conclude that the administrative reforms have been effective. Moreover, the integration of policy measures is also considered to be generally successful. However, none of these studies show the extent to which the social renewal policy has contributed to a reducing the occurrence of social disadvantage in society.

FUTURE PROSPECTS AND STRATEGIES

The widening gap between the rich and the poor

The evidence on the evolution of poverty in the Netherlands clearly suggests that enhanced economic growth does not necessarily imply falling poverty rates and rising economic and social equality. On the contrary, recent evidence shows that the incidence of poverty remains substantial despite economic growth. At the same time, the prevalence of persistent poverty among particular categories, such as the very old, lone mothers, the long-term disabled or unemployed and widows, also remains high. One-out-of-seven people experienced poverty at least once over a six-year period. A large fraction of the population has been prone to persistent poverty, notwithstanding favourable economic conditions. Poverty is clearly present among the Dutch population, not only amongst the lowest income groups but also the middle income groups. Those who were dependent on welfare saw their exit rates from poverty fall because there were less movements into jobs that could raise their income level above the poverty threshold. It might therefore be concluded that increasing persistent poverty rates and income inequality further widened the gap between the fortunate and the socially excluded in society. Although there is a sizeable economic mobility from poverty into non-poverty, particular groups at the lowest end of the income distribution, or with relatively deprived living standards, have little chance of escaping from poverty. Mobility is high among people who are just above, or just below, the income or deprivation poverty thresholds, but low among people in the lower strata.

The decline in relative deprivation

The rise in real incomes of the average worker has gone hand-in-hand with the improvement of the general living conditions. Between 1985 and 1991, the average level of deprivation fell significantly each year. Consequently, the incidence of deprivation-poverty fell during this period, because of the general improvement in living conditions. The evidence suggests that the fall in deprivation-poverty in this period must be attributed to a lower probability of entering poverty rather than a higher probability of escaping from poverty.

The role of the labour market

An important feature of the Dutch labour market has been the rise in employment in atypical or flexible jobs. These jobs are most frequently occupied by married women re-entering the labour market (after a period of withdrawal because of caring duties) and young people entering the labour market for the first time (school-leavers). There is considerable mobility from these flexible jobs into permanent jobs. For people receiving general assistance or unemployment benefit, the likelihood of acquiring a permanent or even a flexible job is extremely low. The longer people receive such benefit, the lower is their probability of entering a permanent or flexible job and thus of escaping from poverty. This implies that long-term poverty and deprivation become more serious even in periods of economic growth. The safety net provided by the general assistance scheme generates little incentives, or opportunity, to escape from poverty. A large fraction of additional earnings are clawed-back from the benefit, which means that the marginal net income gains of any increase in working hours employed are low. Few people are capable of escaping poverty through movements into a job or by changing their household composition by (re)marriage. For most people, even these temporary movements out of poverty are impossible and a persistent dependence on general assistance and a life in poverty remains their only prospects. The threat of rising long-term poverty among people dependent on welfare and social protection in a period of economic upswing gives a strong impetus and legitimisation for social policies that combat social exclusion and increase social cohesion and solidarity.

The role of integrative social policies

Increased social stratification urges for the operation of local, national and transnational policies to combat social exclusion and to foster social integration. At the local level, there is a greater need for integrative policies in order to prevent persistent dependency and to offer schooling, employment and participation opportunities. There is a need for a more flexible and less institutionalised individual approach through active operation of mediating agencies and continuous support through the employment offices to bring the socially disadvantaged back into the labour market or to let them participate in social activities (for example, voluntary associations) or schooling. Intensive and tailor-made mediation activities enabled through new legislation should, according to this view, give greater room for local policies.

In the end, a fundamental reform of Dutch social protection is required to increase job search and to make it more attractive to accept a job and to provide more tools to combat social exclusion.

For the policies to combat social exclusion at the local level it is important that, to avoid treatment differences of individuals, the national authorities should have the primary responsibility to carry out income policies whereas the local authorities should have the responsibility for the execution of schooling, work experience and social activities. The income policy reforms at the national level should raise incentives for the creation and acceptance of jobs, lower unemployment and create opportunities for social participation. The conventional wisdom in the current system of social protection – that receiving a benefit and a wage are purely exclusive events – must be questioned. It then follows that the rate at which benefits are clawed back from earnings is reduced and that the earnings below the hourly minimum wage can be supplemented by a minimum guarantee from general assistance. But it also implies that the different treatment of paid and unpaid labour must be questioned and put into a challenging policy perspective in which there is greater room for policies to bring work that has disappeared back into the market. The rise in labour costs of jobs in the less productive sectors of the economy like the service sector and the public sector (health care, care services, education) together with the cuts in public expenditure spending in the late 1970s and 1980s have led to the disappearance of a large number of jobs in these sectors. By lowering the costs at which these types of jobs can be fulfilled, through lowering the wage-tax bill or a regressive system of wage subsidies, some of these jobs can be recovered. A progressive subsidy scheme means that the subsidy falls with rising wages up to a certain ceiling. By lowering the wage costs not only part of the lost jobs can be recovered but new jobs, particularly in the service sector, may be created. To avoid the negative social effects of it one should keep the former conclusion in mind that earnings below the social minimum must be supplemented to guarantee the minimum living standard. By this proposal part of the jobs which are yet unpaid may again be supplied by the market. However, for many of these unpaid jobs it is very unlikely that these can be transformed into full-paid jobs. For these voluntary jobs, payment cannot be guaranteed through the market. If the provision of these unpaid jobs serve a truly social need, payment, if any, can only be warranted through the public sector. The challenge for public policies is to create new tools for serving these social needs which are better suited to fulfil the desired aims. This may mean a move away from the traditional collective, institutional tools to more functional, flexible and more individualised policy instruments. An example of this exists in the Dutch health care policies, more particularly the so-called 'individual care subsidy'. Older people who are assigned for an old-age home may freely choose to stay at home and to use the care budget for buying the necessary medical and social care services.

Enhanced competition at the international level requires more co-ordination of policy responses at the transnational level, particularly at the level of the European Community, since increased competition will give an advantage to economies with a low level of social protection and a disadvantage to economies with a high level of protection. This could lead to social dumping or a downgrading of social protection levels because of social tourism (movements to states with better social protection) and unwanted migration flows endangering the convergence of social protection systems. The notion of subsidiarity – the guiding principle of the Social Protocol of the Maastricht Treaty – on the one hand and the need for co-ordination on the other hand poses a major challenge for the European Commission to cope with conflicting demands in the social domain.

THE POLICY IMPLICATIONS OF POVERTY RESEARCH

Research reports on poverty made it convincingly clear to policy makers that poverty really exists in the Netherlands. It was only in 1995, after the 'purple' coalition came into force, that a policy report was produced on how to prevent and combat poverty (Netherlands, Second Chamber 1995). Research on poverty in the early 1990s called for particular attention to high levels of poverty, its stability over time and high levels of economic mobility. Less attention was paid to the causes and structural determinants of the processes of impoverishment and social exclusion. The statement in the government report that poverty is primarily an individual and not a societal problem reflects this view. There is growing awareness in the public debate to account for the persistent and long-term character of poverty. This implies for future research that the focus should be on studying the determinants of inflow into and outflow from poverty, the processes of impoverishment-enrichment and social exclusion-integration, its consequences and outcomes, and social policy programmes at the local, national and transnational level.

REFERENCES

Atkinson, A.B. (1987) 'On the Measurement of Poverty', *Econometrica* 55: 749–64.

Bane, M. and Ellwood, D. (1986) 'Slipping Into and Out of Poverty: The Dynamics of Spells', *The Journal of Human Resources* 21 (1): 1–23.

Berghman, J. (1995) 'Social Exclusion in Europe: Policy Context and Analytical Framework', in G. Room (ed.) *Beyond the Threshold: The Measurement and Analysis of Social Exclusion*, Bristol: The Policy Press.

Bosch, K. van den (1994) 'Poverty Measures in Comparative Research'. A paper presented at the Eighth Annual Meeting of the European Society for Population Economics (ESPE), Le Tilburg, The Netherlands, 24 June.

Commission of the European Communities (1994) *Social Protection in Europe*, Luxembourg: Office for Official Publications of the European Communities.

Deleeck, H., van den Bosch, K. and de Lathouwer, L. (eds) (1992) *Poverty and the Adequacy of Social Security in the EC: A Comparative Analysis*, Aldershot: Avebury.

Desai, M. and Shah, A. (1988) 'An Econometric Approach to the Measurement of Poverty', *Oxford Economic Papers* 40: 505–22.

Dirven, H.-J. and Berghman, J. (1991) *Poverty, Insecurity of Subsistence and Relative Deprivation in the Netherlands: Report 1991*, Le Tilburg: Tilburg University.

Dirven, H.-J. and Fouarge, D. (1995) 'Impoverishment and Social Exclusion: A Dynamic Perspective on Income Poverty and Relative Deprivation in Belgium and the Netherlands'. A paper presented at the International Conference on Empirical Poverty Research, Bielefeld, Germany, 17–18 November.

—— (1996) *Income Mobility and Deprivation Dynamics Among the Elderly in Belgium and the Netherlands* (WORC Paper 96.05.005/2), Le Tilburg: Tilburg University, Work and Organisation Research Centre.

Duncan, G.J., Gustafsson, B., Hauser, R., Schmauss, G., Messinger, H.,

Muffels, R., Nolan, B. and Ray, J.-C. (1993) 'Poverty Dynamics in Eight Countries', *Journal of Population Economics* 6 (3): 235–59.

Engbersen, G., Schuyt, K., Timmer, J. and van Waarden, F. (1993) *Cultures of Unemployment*, Boulder: Westview Press.

Engbersen, G., Vrooman, J. C. and Snel, E. (eds) (1996) *Arm Nederland: Het Eerste Jaarrapport Armoede en Sociale Uitsluiting* (Poor Netherlands: The First Annual Report on Poverty and Social Exclusion), The Hague: VUGA Uitgeverij B.V.

Erikson, R., Goldthorpe, J.H. and Portocarero, L. (1979) 'Intergenerational Class Mobility in Three Western Countries: England, France and Sweden', *British Journal of Sociology* 30: 415–41.

Eurostat (1987) *Labour Force Survey: Results 1985*, Luxembourg: Office for Official Publications of the European Communities.

—— (1993) *Labour Force Survey: Results 1991*, Luxembourg: Office for Official Publications of the European Communities.

—— (1995a) *National Accounts ESA 1970–93, Aggregates*, Luxembourg: Office for Official Publications of the European Communities.

—— (1995b) *Social Protection Expenditures and Receipts 1980–93 National Accounts ESA 1970–93, Aggregates*, Luxembourg: Office for Official Publications of the European Communities.

—— (1996) *Labour Force Survey: Results 1994*, Luxembourg: Office for Official Publications of the European Communities.

Fouarge, D. and Dirven, H.-J. (1995) 'Income Dynamics Among the Elderly: Results of an International Comparative Study', *Actes des XVᵉ Journées de l'Association d'Economie Sociale*, Nancy: Berger-Levrault GTI.

Goedhart, T., Halberstadt, V., Kapteyn, A. and van Praag, B.M.S. (1977) 'The Poverty Line: Concept and Measurement', *Journal of Human Resources* 12: 503–20.

Hagenaars, A., de Vos, K. and Zaidi, M. (1994) *Poverty Statistics in the Late 1980s: Research Based on Micro-Data*, Luxembourg: Office for Official Publications of the European Communities.

Lemmens, R.M.M. (1991) *The Socio-Economic Panel Survey: Content, Design and Organisation*, Voorburg/Heerlen: Statistics Netherlands.

Mack, J. and Lansley, S. (1985) *Poor Britain*, London: Allen and Unwin.

Muffels, R. (1993) *Welfare Economic Effects of Social Security – Essays on Poverty, Social Security and Labour Market: Evidence from Panel Data*, Le Tilburg: Tilburg University.

Muffels, R. and Dirven, H.-J. (1995) *Long-term Income and Deprivation Based Poverty. A Comparative Study on the Dutch and German Paneldata* (WORC Paper 95.12.029/2), Le Tilburg: Tilburg University, Work and Organisation Research Centre.

Muffels, R., Dirven, H.-J. and Fouarge, D. (1995) *Armoede, Bestaansonzekerheid en Relatieve Deprivatie: Rapport 1995. De Ontwikkeling van Armoede in Nederland met Bijzondere Aandacht voor de Situatie van Ouderen en Werkenden* (Poverty, Insecurity of Subsistence and Relative Deprivation: Report 1995. The Evolution of Poverty in the Netherlands Focusing on the Situation of the Elderly and the Employed), Le Tilburg: Tilburg University Press.

Netherlands, Second Chamber (1994) *Sociale Nota 1995*, The Hague: Sdu Uitgeverij.

—— (1995) *De Andere Kant van Nederland: Preventie en Bestrijding van Stille Armoede en Sociale Uitsluiting* (The Other Side of the Netherlands: Preventing and Tackling Poverty and Social Exclusion), The Hague: Ministry of Social Affairs and Employment.

Netherlands, Statistics Netherlands (1992) *Statistisch Jaarboek 1992* (Statistical Yearbook 1992), Voorburg/Heerlen: Statistics Netherlands.

—— (1996a) *Statistisch Jaarboek 1996* (Statistical Yearbook 1996), Voorburg/Heerlen: Statistics Netherlands.

—— (1996b) *Maandstatistiek van de Bevolking* (Monthly Bulletin of Population Statistics), 96/1, Voorburg/Heerlen: Statistics Netherlands.

—— (1996c) 'Lage Inkomens 1994' ('Low Incomes 1994'), *Monthly Bulletin of Socio-Economic Statistics* 13, November, Voorburg/Heerlen: Statistics Netherlands.

Organisation for Economic Co-operation and Development (OECD) (1996) *Employment Outlook*, Paris: OECD Publications.

Oeij, P.R.A. (1993) *Combating Social Exclusion in the Netherlands. A Case Study on Social Renewal Policy with Special Reference to Labour Market Policy: Agencies, Institutions and Programs*, Le Tilburg: Institute for Social Research (IVA).

Oorschot, W. van (1991) 'Non-take-up of Social Security Benefits in Europe', *Journal of European Social Policy* 1: 15–30.

Ringen, S. (1988) 'Direct and Indirect Measures of Poverty', *Journal of Social Policy* 17: 351–65.

Roebroek, J. (1993) *The Imprisoned State: The Paradoxical Relationship Between State and Society*, Le Tilburg: Tilburg University.

Sen, A. (1979), 'Issues in the Measurement of Poverty', *Scandinavian Journal of Economics* 81: 285–307.

Serail, S. and Ter Huurne, A. (1995) *Projecten ter Stimulering van de Arbeidsdeelname van Kansarmen in de Regio Noord-Oost Brabant* (Projects Aimed at Increasing Labour Market Participation of the Socially Disadvantaged in the Region of North-East Brabant), Le Tilburg: Institute for Social Research (IVA).

Townsend, P. (1979) *Poverty in the United Kingdom: A Survey of Household Resources and Standards of Living*, Harmondsworth: Penguin.

—— (1987) 'Deprivation', *Journal of Social Policy* 16: 125–46.

Ultee, W., Arts, W. and Flap, H. (1992) *Sociologie: Vragen, Uitspraken en Bevindingen* (Sociology: Questions, Conjectures and Findings), Groningen: Wolters-Noordhoff.

Wouden, R. van der, Ruinaard, M., Kwekkeboom, R., Ter Borg, E., Voogt, P. and Wiertsema, W. (1994) *Evaluatie Sociale Vernieuwing: Het Eindrapport* (The Evaluation of Social Renewal: Final Report), Rijswijk: Social and Cultural Planning Office.

Chapter 8

Philippines

Karen E. Gerdes and Kyle Lynn Pehrson

On the 13 June 1992, Fidel V. Ramos assumed the office of President of the Philippines for one six-year term (1992–8). Ramos was elected by a small minority (only 24 per cent of the vote) in a bitterly contested seven-candidate race. The politico-historical and socio-economic legacy inherited by Ramos was daunting. Four hundred years of colonialism and oppression, widespread persistent poverty since the Second World War, and the martial law years and excesses of the Marcos regime, in which Ramos was a significant player as Chief of the Philippine Armed Forces, had culminated in tremendous socio-economic inequality.

In 1991, just before Ramos took office, 40.7 per cent of the populace was living in poverty. Some analysts argue that the poverty rate was actually 55 per cent. Nine million people were deducted from the poverty count when the government removed a number of basic goods from the traditional 'basket of goods' generally used to determine the poverty line (*Philippine Star* 23 February 1993, p. 5). The richest 20 per cent of the country had a 54.6 per cent share of the national income, while the bottom 40 per cent of the people only had a 13 per cent share (Philippines, National Statistical Coordination Board 1991). Twenty per cent of the population owned 80 per cent of the land (Putzel and Cunnington 1989). While the rich were living in palatial homes, the poor were living in impoverished houses made of scrap wood, metal and cardboard (Putzel 1992).

The enormous socio-economic inequality, fuelled by government corruption and criminality (including human rights abuses, particularly under the authoritarian Marcos regime), had created political instability and spawned a militant communist insurgency, as well as an armed Muslim separatist movement. In reaction, a right-wing militia separated itself from the Philippine Armed Forces after the Marcos years.

Peace and order problems were further complicated by a global recession, natural disasters, a P120 billion trade deficit, and a shortage of arable land (Meyer 1993; Ople 1992). The result was exploding unemployment (15 per cent) and underemployment (20 per cent) (de Dios and Associates 1993), widespread disease (for example, tuberculosis) and environmental degradation. Ramos was now at the helm of one of the world's poorest countries in terms of per capita monthly income (P1,750) (Philippines, National Statistical Coordination Board 1991).

The centrepiece of Ramos' socio-economic strategy was to 'Fight Against Poverty', which he viewed as the key to restoring political stability and social cohesion (Ramos 1993). The purpose of this chapter is to explore and analyse the Ramos administration's response to persistent poverty and socio-economic inequality. We begin with a profile of the country followed by a brief overview of the politico-historical and socio-economic policies of the Philippines that provide a context for the Ramos administration's Social Reform Agenda (SRA). We provide a summary and analysis of current policies and programmes intended to alleviate poverty in the Philippines. Finally, we delineate suggestions to further mitigate poverty in the future.

THE PHILIPPINES: A COUNTRY PROFILE

The Philippines is an archipelago of 7,107 islands situated in the heart of Southeast Asia. The islands are surrounded by the China Sea on the west; the Pacific Ocean on the east; the Sulu and Celebes Seas to the south; and the Bashi Channel to the north. Taiwan, Hong Kong, and China are to the north, while Singapore, Malaysia and Thailand are to the west. The islands of Borneo and Indonesia are to the south-west. The Philippines is a predominantly agricultural country and the majority of the people live in the countryside.

Eleven islands make up 95 per cent of the land area (over 300,000 square kilometres). The majority of the Filipino people inhabit three large island groups: Luzon (141,395 square kilometres, the major city is Manila); Visayas (56,606 square kilometres, the major city is Cebu); Mindanao (101,999 square kilometres, the major city is Davao). These three island groups are further subdivided into fourteen regions, seventy-six provinces, sixty cities, 1,542 municipalities, and 41,825 barangays.

Metropolitan Manila is the national capital region which is composed of the cities Manila (capital), Quezon, Pasay, and Kalookan. Northern Luzon and Mindanao are largely defined along cultural, linguistic, and ethnic factors. For example, Northern Luzon is one of the last strongholds of militant communist insurgents and Mindanao is predominantly Muslim.

One of the country's uniquely decentralised local governments is the Autonomous Region in Muslim Mindanao (ARMM). ARMM allows four provinces (Tawi-Tawi, Sulu, Lanao del Sur and Maguindanao) to have an autonomous regional government. The ARMM is authorised to initiate and attract direct foreign investments for the development and growth of its mainly Muslim population.

The people

Filipinos are of Indo-Malay, Chinese, and Spanish ancestry. The indigenous Negritos probably migrated from Borneo and Sumatra over 30,000 years ago. The national language is Filipino or Tagalog, which is a derivative of Malay if not an actual dialect. There are over 70 other local languages and dialects in the Philippines today. The major languages include Ilocano, Cebuanon and Bicol.

English is understood in many areas but generally only widely spoken among the dominant classes; Spanish and Chinese are spoken by small minorities. The poor and indigenous communities speak in their native languages and are less comfortable with the Western culture and power structures that have been adopted by the rich (Philippines, National Economic and Development Authority (Philippines, NEDA) 1995).

The majority of Filipinos are Catholic (86 per cent), followed by Muslims and Protestants, including a sect that originated in the Philippines called Iglesia ni Kristo. While the Philippines boasts a high literacy rate (93.1 per cent in urban areas; 76.9 per cent in rural areas), communication can still be difficult given the historical, cultural, religious, language and economic diversity in each region.

The Philippines is the world's fourteenth most populated country with approximately 67 million inhabitants. It is also one of Asia's smallest nations in terms of land mass. Therefore, the Philippines has one of the highest population density rates in Asia, an average of 237 people per square kilometre (Garcia 1994). The estimated annual growth rate is 2.8 per cent. By the year 2000, the Philippines is projected to have a population of over 70 million people.

The intense population pressure on a fragile land base is exacerbated by the manner in which the land is controlled and used (Meyer 1993). As the population exponentially increases, the number of non-land-owning agricultural workers continues to expand. Over half of the Filipino population is currently dependent on agriculture, working in rice paddies, cornfields, and cutting sugar cane to provide a living for their families. Agricultural workers or peasants are in a perpetual state of dependence on landowners; therefore, they are unable to make a meaningful contribution to the nation's economic development (Putzel and Cunnington 1989). In addition, the landless rural poor are using forest lands to scratch out a living. Poor fisher folk often resort to dynamiting and other illegal means which may permanently damage the ecosystem (Pineda-Ofreneo 1991). The natural resource depletion, poverty and the pressure it exerts on the environment have already done inestimable damage (for example, illegal logging has resulted in deforestation and flash flooding) (Meyer 1993).

Politico-historical and socio-economic context

Communal land ownership and the spirit of 'bayanihan' or mutual assistance and co-operation was the dominant framework for social welfare in the early Philippines. A '*barangay*' was a small community ruled by a '*datu*' or chief. The people who lived within a certain *barangay* owed their allegiance to the *datu*, not to a tribal or national government. The early Filipinos had their own literature, and social and religious structures (Scott 1994). All indications suggest that commercial ties between China, Arabia, other Islamic merchants and the Philippines existed long before the Spanish came.

Ferdinand Magellan came upon the islands in 1521 and claimed them in the name of King Philip II of Spain. He christened the islands 'Felipinas,' the Philippines. The Spanish brought with them the Catholic religion, a new economic and political system which included private ownership of land – huge land holdings were given to a privileged few – and poverty, which emerged from the introduction of social stratification. Almsgiving and institutional care slowly replaced the communal lifestyle of the *barangays* (Putzel 1992).

Although the Filipinos were a peace loving people they attempted to gain their freedom from the Spaniards through armed rebellion several times. The Philippine people declared their first independence on 12 June 1898. Their independence was short-lived as the Americans took over after the Spanish-American War and introduced Western-style democracy and public education. The Americans also exploited the Philippines for its natural resources, processing them in America and then selling the processed goods back to the Filipino people at a substantial profit (Arcilla 1994). The Japanese occupied the Philippines for a short time during the Second World War. Philippine independence was finally recognised on 4 July 1946.

During the post Second World War period years a 'landed elite' and foreign investors (especially the United States (US)) controlled the Philippine economy. Many of the Philippine export earnings actually went to US multinational companies, while the Philippines remained an exporter of cheap agricultural products like sugar and coconuts (Santos and Lee 1989). An import substitution programme was attempted (that is, Filipino companies tried to make the products that were being imported from the US) for a short period of time. The programme failed because the poor could still not afford to buy the goods and the rich preferred the US imported products (Balisacan 1992).

The Marcos regime: 1962–86

President Ferdinand Marcos promoted an 'import liberalisation, privatisation, foreign loan and an export dependent' economy (Santos and Lee 1989: 7). Poverty deepened despite a modest increase in the average national income. However, growth by the mid-1980s was grinding to a halt. Foreign debt had increased from P40 billion in 1970 to P492 billion in 1983. This led to a tremendous increase in the export of labour (Santos and Lee 1989). Even today, the government continues to support a policy of exporting Filipino labourers to earn foreign currency and solve local unemployment problems. Overseas workers are often subject to serious abuse and exploitation (Ortigas Peace Institute 1993; Pineda-Ofreneo 1991). By the time Marcos was ousted from office in 1986 the foreign debt had grown to P560 billion, the highest in Asia.

The Aquino administration: 1986–92

The 1986 'People Power' revolution that ousted Marcos and swept Corazon Aquino into the office of the Presidency of the Philippines restored democracy, but perhaps more importantly it marked an epiphany in the Filipino consciousness. Empowerment was now more than just a word. The Aquino government re-established and improved upon the Philippine Constitution that Marcos had trampled. The 1987 Constitution provided for a democratic and republican state with a presidential form of government. Legislative (a twenty-four member Senate and a 250 member House of Representatives) and judicial (the Supreme Court) branches of government were designed to ensure adequate checks and balances on presidential powers.

Perhaps more importantly, in 1991, the Aquino government passed the Local Government Code which instituted decentralised and autonomous local government units allowing provinces, cities, municipalities and *barangays* to develop their own socio-economic base through self-initiative and internally-generated revenue schemes. This devolution of powers and funds from the national government to local governments (Nebres 1995) benefited *barangays* and municipalities most, while the provincial governments actually lost some powers.

Despite the above successes, the Aquino government was largely ineffectual in reducing poverty and the foreign debt. When Aquino took office she promised the International Monetary Fund (IMF) and World Bank that the Philippines would honour the debts the Marcos regime had accrued, even though some of the debt involved fraudulent practices (for example, the Bataan Nuclear Power Plant). Aquino relied on the IMF and the World Bank because she believed the only way to improve the economy was through foreign capital (Miranda 1988).

Power shortages between 1990 and 1992 often immobilised the country and therefore the economy. Aquino was also hampered by a series of national disasters. A drought in 1986 had caused damage of P430 million. During the 1990s, Bohol, Region IV and four regions of Luzon were damaged by earthquakes (the estimated damage was P12.3 billion). The last blow was in 1991, when the volcano Mount Pinatubo erupted, completely changing the landscape in Region III and resulting in another P12 billion in damage (Philippines, NEDA 1995). Lastly, Aquino's promises of major agrarian reform and land redistribution never really materialised.

The Ramos administration: since 1992

When elected, Ramos defined his priorities as follows: to restore political and civic stability; to nurse the economy back to health and restore it to growth (for example, dismantle an oligarchic economy with monopolies and cartels); to address the problem of crime and corruption; and to reduce poverty. Ramos dubbed his strategic framework 'Philippines 2000'.

Halfway through his six-year term, is Ramos on course with Philippines 2000? A picture of President Ramos appeared on the cover of the 15 May 1995 edition of Asia's *Time* magazine, with the heading, 'Looking Up: The no-nonsense leadership of Fidel Ramos is energising the Philippines'. The Gross National Product (GNP) has steadily increased since Ramos took office in 1992 with a record performance of 5.5 per cent growth in GNP in 1994, and projections for 6.2 per cent in 1995 and 7.3 per cent in 1996 (Arroyo 1995). For the first time in 20 years the government had achieved a budget surplus. Investments grew. Capital from the country's top ten investors increased 300 per cent from 1993 (Anonymous 1995a).

Peace and order problems are still an issue. Ramos's 1993 Unification Commission, however, utilised a massive consultation process, the most broadly based ever undertaken, to address the people's issues. The process has only begun, but for the first time many parties feel 'heard'. The mid-term election (on 8 May 1995) success of Ramos' Lakas-Laban coalition party is another indicator of the people's confidence in the Ramos government. Nine of twelve available Senate seats went to Lakas-Laban candidates.

However, critics of Ramos are quick to point out the surface level of Ramos's early successes. The increase in the GNP was due largely to a 14.3 per cent growth in electricity due to the establishment of power plants to halt the prolonged brown-outs that plagued the Aquino administration, and a 9.4 per cent increase in construction due to speculative real estate and infrastructure projects (IBON Philippines Databank 1994a). Crispin Beltran, the chairperson of the Kilusng Mayo Uno (KMU, one of the Philippines' largest labour unions), declared that during the first two years of the Ramos administration the gap between the rich and poor had only

widened because of 'bias towards foreign interests rather than the
Filipino people' (KMU International 1994). In fact, there has been
no decline in unemployment, the trade deficit is widening and there
are questions about the sustainablity of the type of growth that has
been promoted by the Ramos administration.

In other words, the macroeconomic growth that has occurred
during the first half of Ramos' term has not yet trickled down to
the poor. Those that have benefited so far are people that already
control capital and are already affluent. The poor remain poor.
Agriculture has been left out of the plans for macroeconomic
growth, the corn and coconut farmers' situations have not improved
(Nebres 1995). In fact, neglect of the rural agricultural sector has
resulted in impoverished farmers migrating to city slums (Arroyo
1995).

Future short-term economic performance is tied to investor
confidence, not a strong export base (Navarro 1995b). Labour, a
vital component of any modernising economy, has thus far largely
been ignored (for example, the number of jobs created in 1994 was
15 per cent less than in 1993). Unemployment continues to increase
(Anonymous 1995b). Thirty per cent of the budget allocation for
1995 was scheduled for debt service (estimated total debt was P680
billion – per capita each Filipino owes P11,320) – while only 2.4
per cent had been allocated for health care (IBON Philippines
Databank 1994a; KMU International 1994).

DEBT, DEVELOPMENT AND POVERTY ALLEVIATION

The socio-economic factors described above are critical to understanding the context of Ramos' current policies to alleviate poverty.
There are basically two schools of thought among social scientists
and economists in the Philippines regarding the relationship
between debt, development, and poverty alleviation. One school of
thought views development and poverty alleviation as mutually
exclusive and debt as destructive (Pineda-Ofreneo 1991; Santos and
Lee 1989). The second school of thought believes macroeconomic
development is a necessary, but not sufficient, means of poverty alleviation, and debt is a natural and acceptable part of development
(Balisacan 1995a).

Early studies indicated that growth strategies in developing
countries actually reduced the income of the poor, especially when
expatriate exploitation of rich natural resources was a part of the

growth strategy (Adelman and Morris 1973; Hollis 1976). Miranda (1988) agreed that macroeconomic growth may actually increase socio-economic inequality that already exists. In fact, Hollis (1976) found that the income of the poorest 60 per cent declines in a growth economy, as does the income of the middle 20 per cent to a lesser degree, while the income of the top 5 per cent increases dramatically. The only way to eliminate inequities is to significantly redistribute assets and increase domestic growth (for example, the development of the agricultural sector so the Philippines can feed itself).

Pineda-Ofreneo (1991) identified five ways in which foreign debt is destructive to the Philippines. First, the outflow for debt robs people of resources for social services. Second, new taxes are sometimes needed, and they often disproportionately affect the poor and lower middle class. Third, the continuing export of Filipino labour to help pay the debt exposes Filipinos to loneliness, exploitation and oftentimes serious abuses by their foreign employers. Fourth, debt increases unemployment because the government cannot create new jobs. The current debt service is the equivalent of paying three million people a minimum wage, or building infrastructure such as schools, hospitals, or accelerated agrarian reform. Finally, the IMF strategy for debt service is anti-union because it requires a pool of cheap labour. Cheap labour is the only advantage the Philippines currently has for competing in the world market. Finally, and more dramatically, Pineda-Ofreneo (1991) claims that limiting the debt service to 20 per cent, instead of the current 30 per cent, could save the life of one Filipino child every hour.

In contrast, Balisacan and Bacawag (1995), among others (Navarro 1995a), believe that macroeconomic development is necessary, if not crucial, to alleviate poverty and that the national debt is not a serious problem as long as the economy continues to grow. Balisacan and Bacawag's (1995: 52) analysis and simulation indicated that if the Philippine GNP continues to grow or stabilises at a per capita growth of about 4 per cent it will take about 12 years for the average poor person to cross over the poverty line:

> Thus, even with growth, it takes a long time – and, for some groups in the society, a lot of pain – to win the war on poverty. But there is no easy alternative. Efforts aimed at promoting and sustaining economic growth induce far more poverty reduction

than any direct, untargeted intervention schemes proposed in recent years (for example, food and credit subsidies).

It has also been argued that economic growth is more productive than offering the rural poor land tenancy alone. However, economic growth must also be accompanied by an improvement in access to social services for the poor (Balisacan 1995b; Balisacan and Bacawag 1995).

Ramos is trying to straddle both of the above viewpoints by first having focused on macroeconomic growth, and now undertaking a very ambitious Social Reform Agenda to help alleviate poverty. While some question the sincerity and unity within the Ramos government, the government has promoted the belief, or at least acknowledged, that macroeconomic growth does not automatically lead to equitable distribution.

In 1994, the government held a Social Reform Summit to seek a balance between global competitiveness and people empowerment. The result of that summit was a comprehensive, integrated approach to poverty alleviation, which will be explored later in the chapter. First, we must define poverty and identify the poor. Then we can undertake a discussion of how best to alleviate poverty.

THE CONCEPT OF POVERTY IN THE PHILIPPINES

On 18 August 1992, President Ramos established the Philippines' Presidential Commission to Fight Poverty (PCFP), citing mass poverty as the principal problem confronting the Philippines today. The PCFP was funded by a grant from the United Nations. The mandate of PCFP was to formulate a comprehensive programme to address the poverty problem and design innovative ways to solve it (Executive Order No. 12 1992). The objectives of the Commission were: to initiate, co-ordinate, integrate, monitor, evaluate and communicate to the public the government's efforts in poverty alleviation; to ensure that these efforts result in the empowerment of people's groups toward self-reliance; and to prepare a blueprint plan of action for a national poverty alleviation effort (Bantilan 1994).

In 1994, the PCFP defined poverty as 'a lack or a deprivation in relation to a social standard' (Philippines, PCFP 1994: 2); in other words, the inability of a household to meet its basic needs for food, clothing, shelter and health care. The PCFP maintains that the government has a responsibility to facilitate a household's ability to sustain itself, either directly or indirectly.

Callanta (1988: 3) provided a similar definition: 'The poor are those whose incomes barely maintain their physical existence and those who have limited or no means of access to other social needs.' Callanta (1988) also identified three ways to operationalise the definition of poverty:

- *Relative poverty* is measured by the income share of the lowest 20 to 40 per cent of the population. (In 1983 the Philippines utilised the bottom 30 per cent of the population to identify those living in relative poverty.)
- *The perception of the people* is measured through the use of self-report scales that generally utilise questions like, 'what do you consider to be the minimum income level needed to maintain a non-poor lifestyle?' (In a 1985 study by the Bishop's Conference, 74 per cent of all Filipinos considered themselves poor, another 13 per cent saw themselves as borderline.)
- *Absolute poverty* is measured in terms of an income level necessary to meet specified minimum nutritional and other basic needs or services (Balisacan 1993; Johansen 1993; Meyer 1993). (A poverty threshold is determined and a headcount is made of those below the threshold.)

In 1983, the Social Development Committee (a Cabinet-level policy-making body) decided to use a relative poverty measure, targeting the bottom 30 per cent with welfare and anti-poverty programmes (Africa 1990). This decision was widely criticised as having 'rendered the extent of poverty vague and therefore almost tantamount to being useless from the viewpoint of planning and programme implementation' (Technical Working Group on Poverty, cited in Africa 1990: xxiii).

The problem with utilising the poor's perceptions to define poverty is that some may accept their fate; and therefore, do not consider themselves to be poor. On the other hand, there may be some people who are hard to please and even though they are not really poor they may consider themselves poor. This does not mean the perceptions of the people should not be considered, but it may not be the best measure of poverty (Balisacan 1992).

The PCFP (Philippines, PCFP 1994: 2) decided to consider what people are constitutionally entitled to; thus, they adopted the absolute poverty threshold as 'the officially determined minimum income needed by a family to obtain a specific bundle of privately provided food and basic services'. The PCFP (Philippines, PCFP 1994) defined basic services as health care, a safe dwelling, clean water and sanitation, and clothing. The food threshold is calculated by determining the minimal nutritional basic requirements (at least 2,000 calories a day, with up to 90 per cent of the calories derived from grains) (Philippines, NEDA 1995).

However, the PCFP is quick to point out the major criticism of the absolute poverty threshold. The basic services component of the absolute poverty threshold is based on what poor people 'actually or typically' spend, not on what they *should* spend. The result is an underestimate of the threshold which results in a very conservative estimate of households in poverty. In addition, when utilising a threshold or cut-off point to measure poverty, a poor person may become poorer but the measured poverty will stay the same (Balisacan 1995a).

The Philippines National Statistical Coordination Board (1991) last determined a *national* absolute poverty threshold in 1991. A family of six (the average number of children in the Philippines is 4.5 per family) would have had to earn more than P3,675 per month or P44,100 a year to be above the poverty threshold. However, in 1991 the poverty threshold for a family of six living in Metro Manila was P5,821 a month (Sarmienton 1991). In 1995, the daily minimum wage in Metro Manila is P145 ($5.80) per eight hour day or P2,900 a month. Since the cost of living has increased substantially since 1991 (thus the poverty threshold when recalculated will also have increased) each household requires several wage earners to stay above the poverty threshold.

INCIDENCE OF POVERTY

Poverty incidence in the Philippines varies widely between 40 per cent to 70 per cent of total households. The variation is, in part, due to disparate conditions in different regions of the country such as prices and services, and temporary factors such as natural disasters (Callanta 1988; McGurn 1990). The variation is also a reflection of a development strategy that generates a highly unequal distribution of income and growth opportunities. For example, the National Capital Region (NCR) and the Visayas witnessed a decrease in poverty between 1985 and 1991 (14.9 per cent of the people living in the NCR were below the poverty line) (Garcia 1994), whereas, Mindanao experienced very little change (Intal 1994). Over 50 per cent of the populations in Northern Western, and Central Mindanao are still living in poverty (Garcia 1994).

Bicol is the poorest region, with 56 per cent of its population living in poverty, despite the fact that it has some of the most fertile soil in the nation (Anonymous 1995a). There are five prominent families in the Bicol region who dominate the economy and who own most of the land. Disproportionate services also dramatically affect the Bicol region. For example, the National Food Authority Statistics (1995) indicate that the National Capital Region includes only 0.3 per cent of the total poverty in the Philippines; however, the NCR has a 22.3 per cent share of the rice. While 13.4 per cent of the nation's poverty is found in Bicol, the region only has 6.4 per cent of the rice distribution. This is, in part, explained by the strong lobbies in the NCR, and the lack of political opposition to the dominant families in the Bicol region.

The lack of political opposition is demonstrated by Representative Edcel Lagman's statement (Anonymous 1995a: 7):

> Bicolanos are so poor, that election day is always payday, since bribe-taking is a way of life . . . . Since people are not politically mature; personal charisma and organisation will carry the day. Incumbents will have a definite edge in 1995.

In addition, Bicol has no infrastructure or skilled human resources to attract investors. Clearly, there is a need to improve access to infrastructure and education to substantially reduce intra-regional poverty in some areas. However, studies indicate that reducing income gaps between regions will only reduce poverty inequity by 20 per cent. By comparison, raising the income of people living within the same region to the mean for that region, may reduce income inequity by as much as 80 per cent (Philippines, NEDA 1995: 47)

The incidence of poverty is higher in rural areas than in urban areas. According to the Ortigas Peace Institute (1993), 60 per cent of Filipinos reside in rural areas and 72.5 per cent of rural families live below the poverty line. Most of the poorest 30 per cent of all households are in rural areas. The Ortigas Peace Institute (1993: 48) attributes most of the rural poverty to skewed land ownership, backward agricultural technology, unavailability of credit, lack of basic physical infrastructure and post-harvest facilities, and over-dependence on foreign markets.

Forty per cent of urban families are poor and live in squatter colonies or slums. The urban poor are constantly threatened by demolitions and relocations. The Ortigas Peace Institute (1993) cites unemployment, under-employment and low income as the cause of urban poverty. Only 84.9 per cent of the urban workforce is employed (and 33.2 per cent of the employed are under-employed or without adequate income), while 15.1 per cent are unemployed (Ortigas Peace Institute 1993).

WHO ARE THE POOR?

Intal (1994: 8–9) identified five important characteristics of poor families:

- *Little or no education*: more than half of all households whose head have no education or at best an elementary education are poor (this includes 75 per cent of all subsistence households). Households whose head have a college education are virtually non-poor.
- *Head aged under 50:* households headed by a person under 50 have a higher incidence of poverty than older households. The lack of remunerable employment for younger people may account for this.
- *Large size*: larger households have a higher incidence of poverty. Seven-member households have a poverty rate of 52 per cent, nine-member households a 60.8 per cent poverty rate.
- *Male-headed*: households with male heads have a much higher-poverty rate than female-headed households! This is perhaps due to higher educational attainment among women and a female-biased employment in the export sector.
- *Subsistence farmers*: most of the subsistence households are farmers, primarily rice, corn and coconut farmers.

The Ramos administration has targeted two poverty groups and five marginalised sectors (Philippines, NEDA 1995: 15–25).

The rural poor

Landless rural agricultural workers or peasants

There are primarily seasonal sugarcane, rice, corn and coconut farmers who neither possess the land they work on, nor do they have officially recognised rights to farm the land. Their average monthly income is only P417.

Marginal upland farmers

These farmers grow rice, corn and other root crops on hills or steep mountain slopes, often in eroded and depleted soil (Callanta 1988). The vast majority earn less than P10,000 a year. They have little access to education and health care and often have no safe water supply.

Cultural communities (indigenous groups)

These are the original settlers of the upland areas whose primary sources of income include subsistence farming, food gathering, fishing and hunting. The Mindanao Lumads, the Cordillera people, the Caraballo tribes, the Negritos of Zambales, the Dumagats, the Mangyans of Mindoro and the Palawan hill tribes combine to make the largest single poverty group (6.7 million people).

Artisans or sustenance fisher folk

Fisher folk, unlike commercial fisherman, use fishing gear that does not require a boat, or else use a small outrigger known as a *banca* (Callanta 1988). Women make up at least 40 per cent of the fisher folk industry. Their contributions range from fish vending to net making and working in fishponds. Incomes earned from fishing range from P3,666 to P8,000 a year (Philippines, NEDA 1995).

Small farm owners – cultivators

Unlike peasants, small farm cultivators own the land they till or have recognised rights to work the land. Their principal produce is rice but they also grow sugarcane and coconuts. In 1990, Balisacan reported that the average annual income of sugarcane farmers was approximately 30 per cent below the poverty threshold. Most coconut farmers live in Mindanao and have been negatively impacted by the Philippines declining share in the global coconut products market.

Small-scale miners

Small-scale miners are found predominantly in Mindanao and work in the vicinity of existing mining concessions or in areas known to have mineral deposits. It is estimated that as many as 63 per cent of small-scale miners live in poverty.

The urban poor

Scavengers

Scavengers can earn between P50 to P100 a day collecting waste products like paper, plastic, and bottles for recycling. Many scavengers live in makeshift huts right on dumpsites. They are often rural migrants who have no education or other skills.

Hawkers, pedlars and micro entrepreneurs

Most hawkers are women under the age of 30. They peddle goods (for example, chewing gum, cigarettes, newspapers) among vehicular traffic or on sidewalks. Because hawkers have no licence to operate they are often the target of police who confiscate their goods. Most hawkers do not earn enough to live above the poverty level.

Union labourers, sweatshop workers

These workers are predominantly young males between the ages of 26 and 35. They generally work long hours for minimal pay, often less than the daily minimum wage. Many live in slum areas and are well below the poverty level.

Marginalised sectors

These include the following groups.

Children in especially difficult circumstances

These include children who are disabled, children of indigenous communities and children of the urban poor. They are plagued by high mortality rates, communicable diseases and malnutrition.

Children who work

Approximately 1.7 million children between the ages of 7 and 14 must work to eke out a living for themselves and/or their families. These children generally receive lower wages than adults for doing comparable work. Most of these children work in rural areas.

Street children

These children are predominantly urban dwellers who were born in slums, and who often have parents who neglected or abused them. They range in age from 6 to 17. There are more males than females in this category. Despite long work hours street children generally earn less than P20 a day. Children who are sexually exploited may earn from P100 to P500 a day. This money is most often shared with families which range from six to eleven people (Garcia 1994).

Prostitutes

Some women in desperate circumstances resort to prostitution to support themselves. In 1985, it was estimated that there were almost 200,000 female prostitutes in the Philippines (Garcia 1994). Since poverty has increased since 1985, it is almost certain the number of prostitutes has grown as well. These women's lower level of skills and education put them at risk. In addition, many Filipino women with an education must resort to taking domestic helper jobs in the Middle East (for example, Saudi Arabia), Hong Kong or Singapore where they may be exploited sexually and/or abused, overworked and underpaid.

Disaster victims

The Filipino people are vulnerable to typhoons, earthquakes, flooding and volcanic eruptions. Every year thousands of families are displaced due to these natural disasters.

The disabled

It is estimated that there are at least 6.5 million disabled persons in the Philippines, including the mentally ill. In 1992 a Magna Carta for Disabled Persons was signed. It provided a framework for delivering services to those in rural areas as well as urban centres. However, services are poor and the disabled tend to be isolated from the rest of society. Many rely on begging to survive.

SOCIAL WELFARE RESPONSE TO POVERTY: THE SOCIAL REFORM AGENDA

In the past, the Philippine Department of Social Welfare and Development (DSWD) has focused its services on marginalised populations, such as, street children, disadvantaged families, youth offenders, teenage mothers, the elderly and disabled. The DSWD continues to remain seriously under-funded. In 1989, only P880 per capita was spent on the poor (Pineda-Ofreneo 1991). Other problems the DSWD have encountered include top-down planning which has resulted in programmes that have not matched the needs of the poor; poor integration and co-ordination with other government agencies, such as the Departments of Health and Education, resulting in a fragmented patchwork of programmes; poor linkages between national government offices and local government offices; and, grossly inadequate access to resources (or poor delivery mechanisms) among low income families, especially in rural areas (Virtucio 1994). Lack of access to basic services has resulted in the following scenario: only 15 per cent of the Philippine population have sanitary sewage systems; 40 per cent of the population have no access to potable water (31 out of 100,000 Filipinos die of preventable water-borne and water-connected diseases each year); and, perhaps as much as 70 per cent of the population is malnourished (Pineda-Ofreneo 1991).

In an attempt to rationalise and integrate social services for the poor the PCFP utilised a grassroots, bottom-up approach and held six regional consultation conferences with the poor and their service providers, including government organisations (GOs), non-government organisations (NGOs), and people's organisations (POs). The six regional conferences culminated in a national workshop to devise a holistic and collaborative strategy to meet the basic needs of the poor.

The result of the national workshop was a three point agenda for social reform (SRA) which focused on the minimum basic needs (MBN) of individuals and families. These were improve access to basic services: *survival* (for example, potable water, health care, education); improve access to economic opportunities and productive resources: *security*; and, more effective participation in economic and political governance: *empowerment*. The goal of the programme is to extend people's capabilities sufficiently to meet their minimum basic needs. Through the SRA, Ramos hopes to reduce poverty from 40 per cent in 1991, the year before he took office, to 30 per cent in 1998 – the end of his six-year term.

The SRA intends to address the basic inequities in Filipino society through a systematic, unified and co-ordinated process referred to as MBN. The nineteen poorest provinces were selected as pilot cites for the MBN programme. Implementation began at the end of May 1995. Table 8.1 identifies the ten minimum basic needs and the twenty-six indicators that those needs are being fulfilled.

Implementation of the MBN programme requires collaborative efforts between the private sector (labour and business), NGOs, POs representing the different poor sectors (peasants, fisher folk), local government representatives (provincial, cities, municipalities and barangays), as well as the following GOs: Department of Agriculture, Department of Environment and Natural Resources, Department of Labour and Employment, Department of Social Welfare and Development, Department of Interior and Local Government, Department of Trade and Industry, Department of Finance, Land Bank of the Philippines, and Housing and Urban Development Coordinating Council.

Ramos issued an Administrative Executive Order to restructure the above-mentioned GOs to focus on the MBN programme and collaborate with each other in the implementation of the programme. There are eight Flagship Programmes (each aimed at a specific sector of the poor) to be implemented by the GOs in co-ordination with the MBN programme: Agricultural Development; Fisheries and Aquatic Resources Conservation, Management and Development; Protection for Ancestral Domains; Workers' Welfare and Protection; Socialised Housing; Compressive Integrated Delivery of Social Services; Institution Building and Effective Participation in Governance; and Livelihood.

To explore how these Flagship Programmes work the sixth programme is used as a case study. Table 8.2 identifies some of the objectives, indicators for success, and the agency responsible for delivery of services under the Flagship Programme: Comprehensive Integrated Delivery of Social Services Flagship Programme.

MBN programme technical groups have been formed at the local level (*barangays* within the targeted nineteen provinces). Each technical group consists of representatives from GOs, NGOs, and POs. The first step for the technical groups has been to develop a community poverty map using the instrument in Table 8.1 to identify the neediest families in each barangay. Initial priority is given to the neediest families. If the situations of the identified families do not change, Ramos intends to hold the top Cabinet Secretaries of the GOs accountable.

How will the Ramos government pay for the ambitious MBN programme? Each national agency concerned will use their appropriated funds to support their respective parts of the programme. In addition, Official Development Assistance (for example, foreign aid in the form of bilateral agreements), United States Agency for International Development (USID), the World Bank and other financial institutions will provide loans and grants. The first stage of the MBN programme is simply to increase access to services. Once that is accomplished the quality of the services can be evaluated. It will be some time before a determination can be made as to the success of the programme.

ANTI-POVERTY PROGRAMMES

Agrarian reform

Agrarian reform refers to programmes that have the intention of redistributing agricultural land to the peasants who till the land, but have no secure access to the land. They, therefore, have no financial security (Putzel 1992). Since the US displaced Spain in 1898 as the coloniser, peasant movements, most recently the military arm of the communist party, the New People's Army (NPA), have periodically erupted to force the issue of agrarian reform.

Putzel (1992) identifies two approaches to agrarian reform: conservative and liberal. The conservative approach, which has steadily been backed by the US, has tended to minimise the distribution of lands belonging to the landed elite. A free market mentality predominates, and the focus changes from land redistribution to problems of low productivity. In contrast, the liberal

Table 8.1 Ten minimum basic needs and their success indicators

Basic needs	Success indicators
A Survival	
1 Food and nutrition	1 Newborns with birthweight of at least 2.5 kg
	2 No severely and moderately underweight children under 5 years old
	3 Pregnant and lactating mothers provided with iron and iodine supplements
	4 Infants breast fed for at least 4 months
2 Health	5 Deliveries attended by trained personnel
	6 Infants 0–1 years old immunised
	7 Pregnant women given two doses of Tetanus Toxoid
	8 No family member gets sick of diarrhoea
	9 No deaths in the family (within the year)
	10 Couples practising family planning.
3 Water and sanitation	11 Family with access to potable water (tap/deep well) within 250 m (10 min. walk)
	12 Family with sanitary toilet (water-sealed, antipolo, flush)
4 Clothing	13 Family members with basic clothing (at least three sets of external and internal clothing)
B Security	
5 Shelter	14 Housing durable for at least 5 years
6 Peace and outer/public safety	15 Family members safe from crimes against person (murder, rape, abuse, physical injury)
	16 Family members safe from crimes against property (burglary theft)
	17 No family members affected by natural disaster
	18 No family member is a victim of armed conflict
7 Income and livelihood	19 Head of the family employed
	20 Other members of the family aged 21 and above employed
C Enabling	
8 Basic education and literacy	21 Children 3–5 years old attending day care/preschool
	22 Children 6–12 years old in elementary school
	23 Family members 10 years old and above able to read and write
9 People's participation in community development	24 Family members involved in at least one people's organisation/association/community development
	25 Family members able to vote at elections
10 Family care/ psycho-social	26 No children below 18 engaged in hazardous occupation

Source: Philippines, PCFP 1994.

Table 8.2 Highlights of the comprehensive integrated delivery of social services Flagship Programme: objectives, indicators of success and agency responsible for delivery of service

Objective	Success indicators	Agency
(1) Basic education		Department of Education, Culture and Sports
All school age children have access to basic education	Number of pupils enrolled	
Elementary school in every *barangay*	Number of *barangays* without elementary school	
High school in each municipality	Number of science laboratory workshops	
	Number of high school teachers needed	
Literacy programme	Literacy rate at *barangay* level	
(2) Community Health Development Programme		Department of Health
	Capacity of POs for planning/managing community resources strengthened	
	Community partnerships between local government and NGOs	
Community-based food supplementation	Procurement of foods	
	Growth charts procured and distributed	
(3) Communal irrigation projects		Department of Agrarian Reform
Road construction, bridge construction, divet lending	Number of irrigation systems per 11.84 km^2	
	Number of road construction or rehabilitation projects in 62.8 km	
(4) Development or capability building programme within local governments		Department of Interior and Local Government
	Capability and competency in mobilising sustainable support for the Philippine Action Plan for children Improved peace and order conditions	
(5) Responsible parenthood services	Number of couples of child-bearing age who received family planning services	Department of Social Welfare and Development
Assistance to individuals in crisis	Number of *barangays* providing financial assistance	
Day care service	Number of *barangays* providing assistance in putting up day care centres	

Table 8.2 Highlights of the comprehensive integrated delivery of social services Flagship Programme: objectives, indicators of success and agency responsible for delivery of service (continued)

Health educational assistance	Number of women who purified water
	Number of women who facilitated construction of a sanitary toilet
	Number of women who cultivated herbal plants
	Number of women who had children immunised
Child placement and protective services	Number of children placed in foster or adoptive homes
Utilising Grameen Bank	Amount of capital funds released to women beneficiaries
Social mobilisation for persons with disabilities	Number of children with signs and symptoms of disabilities provided with intervention services
	Number of day care centres for elderly improved or expanded

Source: Philippines, Social Reform Summit 1994.

approach has supported land redistribution as the most effective way to avoid an all-out revolution.

Proponents of a radical approach to agrarian reform have focused on the landed elite or land monopoly as the greatest obstacle to rural development (IBON Philippines Database 1994b). Radical true believers have also pushed for increased accessibility to financing, and technical and market aid.

In 1987 Aquino initiated the Comprehensive Agrarian Reform Program (CARP), which targeted 103,000 square kilometres of land for redistribution, mostly idle, abandoned, or government-owned lands, of which some 30,000 square kilometres were identified as private lands. However, within the Philippines today 7,000 square kilometres are currently owned by the landed elite (Valencia 1994). The Aquino administration aligned itself with a conservative approach to agrarian reform, and did not place enough emphasis on access to credit, expertise, and technology (Nebres 1995). As a result, when Ramos took over from Aquino in 1992 CARP had only reached about 18 per cent of its stated goals for land redistribution.

The Ramos administration has continued CARP and has struggled with some of the same problems encountered by Aquino. Between 1992 and 1994 Ramos only achieved 12 per cent of his administration's targeted goals for land redistribution. CARP has been centralised at the national level with very few delivery mechanisms in place at the local and provincial levels. In addition, there has been a lack of co-ordination between the many agencies responsible for implementing CARP. These include, but are not limited to the Department of Agriculture, the National Irrigation Administration, the Department of Public Works and Highways, the Department of Environmental and Natural Resources, the Land Bank of the Philippines, and the Justice Department.

In May 1995, Ramos began to redistribute lands belonging to the landed elite. However, there have been problems with the mediation mechanism. The few clans who own most of the land, particularly the sugar barons, have not voluntarily given up any land. An initial land valuation is done by the Land Bank of the Philippines. The land owner may accept or reject the offer. Most land owners reject the offer, and are likely to request a second valuation. The land owners can appeal to the court system if they do not agree with the second valuation. If the court requires the land owner to accept the offer of payment, the land title is then placed in the name of the peasant or farmer. However, having the title in their name does not necessarily mean they can take possession of the land. Many land owners have small militias that threaten or harass new title-holders.

In the near future, the Ramos government hopes to reach an agreement with the Philippine National Police to install small farmers on their new land and protect them from the militias of the landed elite. Another strategy that has recently begun within the administration is to avoid compulsory acquisition of land by asking the land owners to voluntarily surrender parts of their land.

Despite these new efforts, local graft and corruption have often prevented the successful implementation of CARP (for example, local police who have ties to the landed elite). Critics of CARP describe two other major roadblocks: the bureaucracy is too slow; and legislation is continually being passed that waters down the objectives of CARP, so that they are more consistent with a conservative approach to agrarian reform (Valencia 1994).

Balisacan (1993, 1994, 1995a, 1995b) argues that rapid and sustained economic growth and employment generation outside agricultural areas, or off-farm jobs, is the only way to alleviate rural poverty. He cites the falling earnings in agriculture, dwindling agricultural exports and rising food imports as evidence that land reform alone, regardless of how it is implemented, is not sufficient to alleviate rural poverty.

Developing Asian countries, such as Indonesia, Malaysia and Thailand, have had success in alleviating rural poverty by focusing on sustainable macroeconomic growth, investment in basic infrastructure, and a favourable agrarian structure (Balisacan 1995b). However, if the Philippines decides to shift from a predominantly agricultural economy to a modern industrial economy, quality education in rural areas will be critical (Balisacan 1992).

Population management

Filipino women have the highest total fertility rate in the Southeast Asian Region (Garcia 1994). Having many children substantially increases the risk of poverty. For example, for a household with one child the risk of poverty is 44–50 per cent; whereas, for a household with five children it increases to 60–78 per cent (Bauer et al. 1992). Bauer et al. also found that family size restricts educational opportunities for children and limits household savings.

In addition, Lee (1993: 42) points out:

> The population problem in the Philippines is best viewed in the context of the realities that the country finds itself in: pervasive poverty, high rates of unemployment in the face of a rapidly changing labor force, poor education, poor health, and poor nutrition among a large proportion of the populace, and severe constraints on the nation's resources arising from poor economic performance and heavy debt burden.

If the Philippines wants to preserve and improve its fragile ecosystems then the population must be controlled (Meyer 1993).

For the past 20 years the Philippine government, through the Department of Health (DOH), has advocated fertility reduction. Most recently, the DOH has focused on scientific family planning (for example, basal body temperature, cervical mucous method, condoms, birth control pills, inter-uterine device), and responsible parenthood in the larger context of development and total family welfare (Greenspan 1992).

Despite the government's efforts, they have recently had to readjust their aggressive family planning campaign under pressure from Cardinal Jaime L. Sin, the head of the Catholic church in the Philippines, who strongly opposes any type of family planning. In spite of the Catholic church's opposition, NGOs and POs have still been able to achieve moderate success with family planning. The NGOs network of clinics have focused more on 'capacity-building of grassroots structures, value formation, and positive attitude change' (Silvia and Cruz 1989: 10) in conjunction with POs, which has made family planning much more acceptable in rural areas. However, there is still a long way to go before the Ramos government can meet its stated goal in population management. The goal is to reduce population growth, which was estimated to be 2.21 per cent in 1993, to 1.92 per cent by 1998 (Philippines, NEDA 1995).

Housing

The Philippines is currently experiencing a backlog of 3.8 million housing units (Philippines, NEDA. 1995). In response, Ramos launched *'Sariling Kayod Para Sa Sariling Bahay'* (Earn Your Own House). In the past, the *Pag-Ibig* Housing Fund (housing assistance) has only been open to government employees and privately-owned company employees. Both the government and the corporations pay into the Fund. Ramos has opened the fund to market vendors, *jeepney* drivers (that is, Filipino version of an open-air taxi), craftsman and other self-employed people who wish to make small contributions. The bottleneck now is that there is not enough land to build all the houses that are needed. Medium rise apartment buildings and housing units that can accommodate up to four families may be creative ways to efficiently use the land that is available.

Unfortunately, the *Pag-Ibig* Housing Fund assistance is also open to private developers who want to build low-cost housing. The NGOs would like to see the people's organisations mobilise to build their own housing units, which would be less expensive than if the private sector constructs the units. The paperwork to access *Pag-Ibig* Housing Fund is burdensome and complicated. Private developers have more resources to deal with the bureaucracy than the small POs.

In Cebu, a time and motion study was undertaken by one NGO to calculate the time it takes to fill out paperwork and eventually have access to *Pag-Ibig* Housing Fund assistance. The result is that it takes three months to finally obtain the assistance requested. At a Housing Summit in 1994, urban poor POs proposed a plan that would reduce the decision lead-time to one and a half months. In addition, they would like to see the law that makes 'squatting' a crime repealed. At the very least, relocation of squatters should be a collaborative process with the people. So far, no progress has been made on the POs suggestions or requests.

Non-government organisations

NGOs are currently focusing on addressing the capability building needs of POs. The basic strategy is to identify, develop and support community leaders, and facilitate the mobilisation of the respective constituencies to transform their own communities. Critical to the NGOs' strategy is a continuation and expansion of the 'people-power' revolution that began in 1986. Dineros-Pineda (1992: 264) defines people power as 'collective action of the powerless against an oppressive system'.

Collective action begins in local organisations or POs with the members knowing their rights and exacting accountability from each other and their leaders. The people power consciousness must then be translated into the ballot when there are local, provincial or national elections. In other words, the POs must first learn the democratic process among themselves before they can be expected to play it out on a larger scale.

For example, several POs collectively organised to defeat an entrenched senate incumbent in the May 1995 elections. The POs were successful and their candidate was elected. Now, they must apply pressure to their new senator to be accountable to the wishes of his constituency. Victories like this one among POs lead to confidence and the increased realisation of power.

NGOs have also been very active in helping groups of Filipinos, often women, start small and medium-sized business enterprises. There are many examples, one of the better known is called the Trickle-Up Program. Between 1979 and 1994, working with sixty-three different co-ordinating agencies, the Trickle-Up Program has helped fund 7,847 small businesses. It works by providing a P2,000 conditional grant (that is, a business plan must be presented in writing) in two P1,000 instalments. The average profit was P2,980, 20 per cent of which must be reinvested into the business.

Most business groups in the Philippines (60 per cent of which are female) used the remaining profit to supplement other incomes (Leet and Leet 1994).

Social security

There are two social insurance systems designed to 'protect [workers] against poverty' in the Philippines: the Government Service Insurance System (GSIS), and the Social Security System (SSS). Both systems provide replacement income for retirement, survivors in the event of death, and disability, sickness, and maternity leave (that is, employee compensation). Members of GSIS and SSS are also covered by medicare which covers hospitalisation and other medical needs. The GSIS was created in 1936 for government employees, while the SSS was implemented in 1957 to protect workers in the private sector and those that are self-employed (Philippines, GSIS 1985; Philippines, SSS 1994).

The above identified compensation programmes are in part made possible by the following monthly contributions from employees and employers (Philippines, SSS 1994: 81):

- Retirement Benefits: 8.4 per cent average monthly compensation not exceeding P9,000 with contributions payable by both employer (5.04 per cent) and employee (3.36 per cent).
- Employee Compensation: 2.5 per cent of average monthly compensation not exceeding P3,000 with contributions payable by both employer and employee in equal shares.
- Medicare: one per cent of average monthly compensation not exceeding P1,000 with contributions payable only by the employer.

In addition to replacement income and medical insurance, members of GSIS and SSS are also eligible for educational and housing loans.

FUTURE STRATEGIES TO ALLEVIATE POVERTY

It is clear that government intervention is necessary to alleviate poverty in the Philippines. In comparison to his predecessors, President Ramos has at least created a framework for rational government intervention (for example, the MBN programme). However, it is still unknown whether the government bureaucracy can effectively and efficiently implement the programme.

The macroeconomic policies of Ramos and his predecessors have thus far benefited the middle and upper classes and have had no visible impact on poverty. This is not to say that macroeconomic growth in and of itself is bad, but rather that the government must intervene aggressively to create or generate effective trickle-down or redistributive mechanisms.

For example, the current tax structure in the Philippines extracts 70 per cent of its revenues from indirect taxes (such as sales tax). Thus, Filipinos living in poverty often have a greater tax burden than middle or upper class families proportionate to their respective incomes (Yoingco *et al.* 1994). A study of the distribution of the total tax burden in 1985 indicated that persons making less than P6,000 a year used 11.72 per cent of their income to pay taxes. Filipinos making between P6,000 and P30,000 a year used, on average, only 10.30 per cent of their income to pay taxes (Yoingco *et al.* 1994: 176). One of the fastest ways Ramos can increase domestic resources and income, while at the same time easing the burden of the poor, is to develop and implement a more progressive tax system.

Thirty-nine per cent of the government's budget allocation goes toward salaries for government employees. Throughout the chapter, references have been made to the large government bureaucracy currently operating in the Philippines. As of December 1993, there were 1.2 million government employees, excluding the Philippine National Police, the Department of National Defense, the Economic Intelligence and Investigation Bureau, and the National Intelligence Coordinating Agency (Garcia 1994). It could be argued that the government is justified in sustaining such a large bureaucracy because it is employing people. However, if government services were more streamlined and required fewer employees, some of the revenue used to finance government employee salaries may be better spent on income redistribution programmes (Yoingco *et al.* 1994).

Decentralised poverty alleviation programmes are needed to address the inequities between and within regions. Thus far, the focus on poverty alleviation has been directed at the barangay or national level, respectively the micro and macro levels. The meso (such as, municipal, provincial, and regional) levels have been largely ignored. To address the inequities between regions and within any given region, programme implementation must be manageable at the meso level. In fact, it may actually be more effective at the meso level in terms achieving of broad, sweeping change.

Finally, the government must follow the lead of the NGOs in training POs and other community organisations how to problem solve at the local level, as well as how to translate their 'people power' into political power on election day. The oppressive political system that has dominated the Philippines for hundreds of years can only be changed by the collective will of the Filipino people.

ACKNOWLEDGEMENTS

The authors would like to acknowledge the following for their assistance in collecting and interpreting data: Arsenio M. Balisacan (Associate Professor of Economics, University of the Philippines); Clifford C. Burkely (Head Executive Assistant, Department of Agrarian Reform); Enrico O. Garde (Associate Director, Ateneo Center for Social Policy and Public Affairs); Corazon Juliano-Soliman (Executive Director, Community Organising Training and Research Advocacy Institute); Manolito A. Novales (Executive Director, Presidential Commission to Fight Poverty); Esther M. Pacheco (Director, Ateneo de Manila University Press); Emmanuel C. Torrente (Social Development Staff, National Economic and Development Authority); and Cristy Antonio.

REFERENCES

Adelman, I. and Morris, C.T. (1973) *Economic Growth and Social Equity in Developing Countries*, Stanford, CA: Stanford University Press.

Africa, T.P. (1990) 'Selected Statistics and Concepts used in Philippine Censuses, Surveys and Development Plans', *Journal of Philippine Statistics* 41 (1) (January–March): ix–xxvi.

Anonymous (1995a) 'Bicol Torn by Factionalism', in Hofilena, C. and Gloria, G.M. (eds) *Politik*, Manila: Florentino-Ateneo Center for Social Policy and Public Affairs.

—— (1995b) 'Philippine Situation', in Hofilena, C. and Gloria, G.M. (eds) *Politik*, Manila: Florentino-Ateneo Center for Social Policy and Public Affairs.

Arcilla, J.S. (1994) *An Introduction to Philippine History*, Quezon City: Ateneo de Manila University Press.

Arroyo, D.M. (1995) 'The Philippine Economy turns the Corner', *Intersect* 9 (1) (January): 4–5 and 18.

Balisacan, A.M. (1992) 'Rural Poverty in the Philippines: Incidence, Determinants, and Policies', *Asian Development Review* 10 (1): 125–63.

—— (1993) 'Agricultural Growth, Landlessness, Off-farm Employment, and Rural Poverty in the Philippines', *Economic Development and Cultural Change* 41 (April): 533–62.

—— (1994) 'Selected Asian Experiences on Agrarian Reform', in *Agrarian Structure and Reform Measures*, Tokyo: Asian Productivity Organisation.

—— (1995a) 'Anatomy of Poverty during Adjustment: The Case of the Philippines', *Economic Development and Cultural Change*.

—— (1995b) 'Agriculture in Transition: Arresting Poverty in the Rural Sector', in Fabella, R.V. and Sakai, T. (eds) *Towards Sustained Growth*, Tokyo: Institute of Developing Economies.

Balisacan, A.M. and Bacawag, R.T.C. (1995) 'Inequality, Poverty, Urban-rural Growth Linkages' (unpublished manuscript), Quezon City: University of the Philippines, School of Economics.

Bantilan, M.S.C. (1994) 'Philippine Poverty Monitoring Systems: Status and Future Directions', in Intal, P.S. and Bantilan, M.C.S. (eds) *Understanding Poverty and Inequity in the Philippines*, Pasig: National Economic Development Authority.

Bauer, J., Mason, A., Canlas, D. and Fernandez, M.T. (1992) 'Poverty in the Philippines: The Impact on Family Size'. A paper presented at the Conference on Priority Health and Population Issues, East-West Center, Manila, 25–8 February.

Callanta, R.S. (1988), *Poverty: The Philippine Scenario*, Makati, Metro Manila: Bookmark.

de Dios, E.S., Medalla, F.M., Gochoco, M.S., Tan, E.A., Jurado, G.M., David, C.C., Ponce, E.R., Intal, P.S., Sanchez, A., Balagot, B.P. and Alburo, F.A. (1993) *Poverty, Growth, and the Fiscal Crisis*, Manila: Philippines Institute for Developmental Studies.

Dineros-Pineda, J. (1992, 'Beyond Nutrition: Empowerment in the Philippines', *International Social Work* 35 (2) (April): 203–15.

Garcia, M.B. (1994) *Social Problems in the Philippine Context*, Metro Manila: National Bookstore Press.

Greenspan, A. (1992) 'Poverty in the Philippines: The Impact of Family Size', *Asia-Pacific Population and Policy* 21 (June): 1–4.

Hollis, C. (1976) *Redistribution with Growth*, London: Oxford University Press.

IBON Philippines Databank (1994a) 'Finally Growth?', *IBON Facts and Figures* 18 (1–2) (January): 2–3.

IBON Philippines Database (1994b) 'Seven Years of Land Reform under the CARP: True Lies', *IBON Special Release* 10 (November): 1–8.

Intal, P.S. (1994) 'The State of Poverty in the Philippines: An Overview', in Intal, P.S. and Bantilan, M.C.S. (eds) *Understanding Poverty and Inequity in the Philippines*, Pasig: United Nations Development Program and National Economic and Development Authority.

Johansen, F. (1993) *Poverty Reduction in East Asia* (Discussion Paper no. 203), Washington, DC: The World Bank.

Kilusng Mayo Uno (KMU) International (1994) 'Two Years under Ramos: The Gap Widens', *Correspondence* 9 (3) (July–August): 1–3.

Lee, A.C. (1993) 'The Quality of Our Lives', *Philippine Panorama* (July): 5–10.

Leet, G. and Leet, M.R. (1994) *1994 Trickle-Up Program Annual Report*, Riverside, NY: Trickle-Up Program.

McGurn, W. (1990) 'Corazon Aquino's Poverty Pimps', *The American Spectator* (September): 14–17.

Meyer, C. (1993) 'Migration Patterns Unravel the Population, Poverty, Environment Tangle', *Development Journal of SID* 1: 12–16.

Miranda, M. (1988) 'The Economics of Poverty and the Poverty of Economics: The Philippine Experience', in Canlas, M., Miranda, M. and Putzel, J. (eds) *Land, Poverty and Politics in the Philippines*, Quezon City: Claretian Publications.

Navarro, N.Y. (1995a) 'The Philippine Economy: An Historical Perspective', *Politik* 1 (4) (May): 16–19.

—— (1995b) 'Prospects for Growth', *Politik* 1 (3) (February): 13–20.

Nebres, B.F. (1995) 'Shifting Trends in the Political Arena', *Intersect*, 9 (1) (January): 6–7.

Ople, B.F. (1992) 'The Philippines after Aquino', *Manila Bulletin* 267 (26) (March 12): 7.

Ortigas Peace Institute (1993), *Basic Peace*, Quezon City, Philippines, Ateneo de Manila University Press.

Philippines, Government Service Insurance System (GSIS) (1985) *A Primer on the Various Types of Social Insurance, Social Security Benefits and Employee Compensation Claims, and the Basic Requirements for Entitlement under the Different Laws as Administered by the GSIS*, Manila: GSIS.

Philippines, National Economic and Development Authority (NEDA) (1995) *Social Development in the Philippines: Vision, Challenges and Imperatives*, Manila: NEDA.

Philippines, National Statistical Coordination Board (1991) *Philippines Statistical Yearbook*, Manila: National Statistical Information Center.

Philippines, Presidential Commission to Fight Poverty (PCFP) (1994) *A Strategy to Fight Poverty*, Manila: PCFP.

Philippines, Social Reform Summit (SRS) (1994) *Program Master Plan of Operations*, a report presented at the Social Reform Summit, September 27, Manila.

Philippines, Social Security System (SSS) (1994) *Guidebook for SSS Members*, Manila, Philippines: SSS.

Pineda-Ofreneo, R. (1991) *The Philippines: Debt and Poverty*, London: Oxfam.

Putzel, J. (1992) *A Captive Land: The Politics of Agrarian Reform in the Philippines*, Quezon City: Ateneo de Manila University Press.

Putzel, J. and Cunnington, J. (1989) *Gaining Ground: Agrarian Reform in the Philippines*, Nottingham: Russell Press.

Ramos, F.V. (1993) 'State of the Nation Address', Second Session, 9th Congress of the Philippines.

Santos, A.F. and Lee, L.F. (1989) *The Debt Crisis: A Treadmill of Poverty for Filipino Women*, Manila: Kalayaan.

Sarmienton, J.V. (1991) 'Metro Family Must Earn P 5,821 Monthly', *Philippine Enquirer* (June 25): 10.

Scott, W.H. (1994) *Barangay*, Quezon City: Ateneo de Manila University Press.

Silvia, T. and Cruz, V.P. (1989) 'Strategic Assessments of NGOs in Population, Family Planning, Health, and Social Welfare', in Quizon, A.B. and Reyes, R.V. (eds) *A Strategic Assessment of NGOs in the Philippines*, Manila: ANGOC.

Valencia, N. (1994) 'Preliminary Assessment of CARP', *Voices From the Grassroots: Report of the National Conference on Land Use Conversion and Agrarian Reform (October 25–8)*, Quezon City: Integrated Rural Development Foundation.

Virtucio, F. K. (1994) 'A Household Survey of the Lowest Income Groups in the Philippines', in Intal, P.S. and Bantilan, M.C.S. (eds) *Understanding Poverty and Inequity in the Philippines*, Pasig: United Nations Development Program and National Economic and Development Authority.

Yoingco, A.Q., Guevara, M.M. and Gracia, J.P. (1994) 'A Study on the Incidence of the Philippine Fiscal System', in Intal, P.S. and Bantilan, M.C.S. (eds) *Understanding Poverty and Inequity in the Philippines*, Pasig: United Nations Development Program and National Economic and Development Authority.

Chapter 9

United Kingdom

Richard Silburn

The extent of poverty in the United Kingdom (UK), its causes and possible remedies have been a topic of intermittent but vigorous public debate since the classic research studies by Charles Booth in London and Seebohm Rowntree in York at the turn of the century (Booth 1903; Piachaud 1987; Rowntree 1901). It is as though poverty becomes an issue of widespread public concern at intervals of about 30 years. Fresh interest in the subject has usually been prompted by the publication of disturbing research evidence; this is greeted with a reaction of widespread distress and shock, which fuels a debate about what appropriate steps should be taken to try to reduce or eradicate poverty. This debate has been made consistently and considerably more difficult, contentious and frustrating by the lack of any official definition of poverty. Indeed, research evidence about poverty has usually provoked governments into a defensive reaction where the accuracy or the significance of the research has been called into question, and the implications for policy are denied or fudged. This marked reluctance to develop or sanction an official definition of poverty, or overtly to build into the policy process any one of the possible definitions suggested by academic enquiry, or, more recently, by one or other of the international or supra-national organisations, has hampered coherent discussion about both the nature and extent of poverty, and appropriate social policies.

If we examine the situation since the end of the of the Second World War, it can be divided into three broad phases. The first, relatively optimistic, phase lasted until the middle 1960s. It was an optimistic period because many people believed that poverty in the post-war UK had been successfully eradicated. The second phase, from the middle 1960s until the end of the 1970s, was of growing concern about the persistence of unacceptable levels of deprivation, as revealed by one of the periodic 'rediscoveries of poverty'. Vulnerable groups in the population were identified, and policy recommendations canvassed. But in the late 1970s the public mood changed again, and the 1979 General Election ushered in a prolonged period of Conservative government disbelieving of, or indifferent to, the plight of the poor, and determined to substitute, wherever possible, market-solutions to social problems. But public confidence in this approach was severely damaged by the economic recession of the late 1980s, and swelling public anxiety about greatly increased social inequality has stimulated a modest revival of concern about poverty as a serious and widespread phenomenon with grave implications for the quality of life of the entire nation.

THE POST-WAR ABOLITION OF POVERTY?

From 1942 onwards, ambitious plans for comprehensive post-war social reconstruction gained widespread public support. The Beveridge Report, published in that year, contained a detailed blueprint for the abolition of what Beveridge described as 'want' (Beveridge 1942). The Beveridge Plan, in intention at least, was accepted by the victorious Labour Government of 1945 and many of its proposals were put into effect by 1948 in a major programme of social legislation which established what came to be known as the welfare state. Acts of Parliament legislated for universal access to health care, free of direct charges at the point of delivery; for a reformed public education system, promising equality of educational opportunity for all; for a social security system, which provided pensions for the elderly, short-term cash benefits for other groups in time of need, and a children's allowance to help families with dependent children; and for a public housing programme, to eradicate urban squalor. But at the heart of the reconstruction process was not an Act of Parliament or law, but a general policy commitment by government to do all in its power to maintain the highest possible level of employment. Full employment was expected to help obliterate the bitter memories of inter-war economic depression by enabling most families first to maintain and then steadily to improve their living standards by their own efforts, with the blessing of a regular income. For a prolonged period in the post-war years full employment was successfully maintained, with the consequence that living standards for the working population and their families improved steadily and visibly. Not surprisingly, it was widely believed, and with some pride, that poverty had been finally eradicated from British society.

Beveridge defined 'want' as the situation where 'families and individuals . . . might lack the means of healthy subsistence' (Beveridge 1942: para. 11). Subsistence was taken to mean something more than brute survival, and included a range of 'human needs', the definition of which reflected changing ideas about what constituted an acceptable standard of living. Here Beveridge relied heavily on the inter-war research work of Seebohm Rowntree, particularly his second survey of poverty in York carried out in 1936, and his book, *The Human Needs of Labour*, in which he tried to specify what an individual or family required in order to maintain 'a healthy subsistence' (Rowntree 1937, 1941). But subsistence remained an austere basis for a definition of poverty, and for establishing the appropriate level to set social security payments or other poverty relief measures. Certainly the new social security system, introduced in 1948, paid pensions and other benefits which were considerably lower than prevailing wage rates, and so could not be seen as sufficient to maintain customary living-standards. But nor were they intended to; the state would only guarantee a basic living standard, to be supplemented by prudent and responsible citizens from private savings and insurances, and by informal and family support networks.

Full employment and rising living standards for most of the working population of working age helped to mask the disadvantaged situation of those who were unable to join the world of paid work. Continuing real hardship was experienced in particular by many elderly people, but even the relatively meagre level of pensions was widely believed, when compared to what had gone before, to have made a genuine if modest improvement in the circumstances of this group too, so confidence in the post-war achievement was not seriously undermined.

It was not until the 1960s that research evidence started to raise serious doubts about the extent of this post-war success. Before this, anxieties were occasionally expressed about the persistence of hardship among some elderly people, particularly those for whom the state pension was the sole source of income (Townsend 1957). The long-continuing housing shortage remained a grievance, and from time to time the deplorable condition of much of the older housing stock was highlighted (Greve 1964). But the belief that in general, and for most people, conditions were getting consistently and considerably better remained dominant.

THE RE-DISCOVERY, AND RE-DEFINITION, OF POVERTY

The publication which reopened the poverty-debate in the mid-1960s and triggered a critical re-evaluation, was an occasional paper by Brian Abel-Smith and Peter Townsend (Abel-Smith and Townsend 1965). They argued not only that poverty was a persistent reality, but also that it had actually been increasing throughout the post-war period, rather than diminishing as was popularly thought. How was poverty defined in this study? For Abel-Smith and Townsend a narrowly defined subsistence standard was plainly inadequate. If living standards were generally improving should not even the poorest have some share of this improvement. In the absence of an official or agreed definition of poverty, Abel-Smith and Townsend argued that means-tested state social assistance payments, based as they were on published, nationally applicable, benefit-scales represented a minimum level of living below which the state would allow no-one to fall. In short benefit levels could be taken as a proxy for an official poverty line. They therefore defined poverty by reference to the levels of means-tested assistance that the social security system offered to those in need. Observing that in addition to basic rates of benefit, successful claimants had their rents paid, and might also be entitled to additional payments for special needs, Abel-Smith and Townsend estimated the numbers of poor households as those with incomes less than 140 per cent of basic entitlement. Although practical, this definition is a limited one; it is a measure of cash-poverty only. It begs the question as to whether these scale-rates are adequate to meet people's needs. But the defining point of poverty was moved pragmatically beyond considerations of subsistence needs. At the time it was a useful and defensible benchmark to start a debate grounded in commonly encountered, real-life circumstances.

Using Abel-Smith and Townsend's definition produced some startling findings. Based upon a re-analysis of Family Expenditure statistics for the years 1954 and 1960, they asserted that the numbers of people living in households with incomes below, or close to, the levels set for means-tested social assistance had been increasing throughout the period, and that in 1960 comprised just over 14 per cent of the population. The groups most likely to be affected were the retired elderly, the sick and disabled, the unemployed (at that time a small number), workers in very low-paid employment, or whose income was inadequate to meet above-average family costs. Abel-Smith and Townsend's work put poverty back on the public agenda, and it remained a key concern throughout the rest of the 1960s and 1970s.

Peter Townsend was clearly dissatisfied with the definition used in *The Poor and the Poorest* and his own continuing work reflects this clearly. In *Poverty in the United Kingdom* (Townsend 1979: 31), he argued for a much broader definition of poverty:

> Individuals, families and groups in the population can be said to be in poverty when they lack the resources to obtain the types of diet, participate in the activities and have the living conditions and amenities which are customary . . . in the societies to which they belong . . . they are in effect, excluded from ordinary living patterns, customs and activities.

The notion of social participation goes beyond measuring patterns of material consumption, to include a wide range of social activities that reflect or confirm an individual's standing within a family, neighbourhood or workplace. Examples might include gift-exchanges within families to mark birthdays or Christmas, or the ability to both give and receive hospitality with friends, neighbours and colleagues. Activities of this kind are driven by custom and social convention modified by personal temperament and taste. To identify poverty with an inability to socially engage in this way, rather than on some narrow list of necessities for survival, encourages a shifting and relative definition sensitive to the changing patterns of daily life.

Townsend argued that poverty defined in this way could be objectively measured, and to this end he developed a 'deprivation index'. This index measured an individual's or family's capacity to participate in a wide range of customary social activities, and, crucially, demonstrated that as family income diminishes so does its social participation. Moreover, Townsend claimed that a critical income threshold is reached beyond which comes an abrupt decline in social participation. In effect, Townsend was suggesting that if it is useful to try to establish a poverty line, then it should be one which reflects the way in which people are able to conduct themselves as active and responsible members of society. Rather than a narrow concern with survival or subsistence needs, Townsend was concerned with the capacity to live a normal life, fashioned by custom and convention, and by widely-shared ideas about social roles and obligations. Townsend's work has been of considerable importance as a major contribution to a more refined academic understanding, but it has had much less impact outside the academy, and this is particularly the case in the world of public policy, where different pressures have been at work.

THE DENIAL OF POVERTY

During the 1970s, and certainly well before 1979, political opinion in the UK was shifting in different directions. The election of the first Thatcher Conservative government in 1979 saw the start of a long period during which market solutions were sought for both economic and social problems. Public expenditure in general, and social welfare expenditure in particular, was perceived as part of the problem rather than part of the solution. The interventionist role of government, in both the economic and the social spheres, diminished. The emphasis shifted to questions of wealth creation rather than its distribution. Official concern about the poor diminished greatly, and the gulf between the academic debate and political responses grew much wider. The government was concerned to push the definition of poverty (if indeed there were any such thing) much closer to an absolute approach, and decisively away from the relative approaches that had been gathering force. By the middle of the 1980s more interest was expressed in the thinking of Charles Murray, and his ideas about a growing 'underclass' of single-parents and long-term unemployed, allegedly corrupted by welfare-benefit dependency and increasingly detached from the mainstream of working society (Murray 1984, 1990). Much less interest was shown in a number of important ideas and new approaches to the definition and measurement of poverty developing within the European Union. In particular, the concept of 'social exclusion', which focused on the processes which marginalise and exclude individuals, families and whole groups. The excluded include not only the cash-poor, but all those who are unable to participate fully in economic, political, social and cultural life (Room *et al.* 1989).

Meanwhile, in common with many other countries, the UK has experienced accelerating changes in the broader economic situation.

The economic and social policies pursued throughout the 1980s, combined with the effects of alternating periods of economic boom and recession, and the increasing impact of changes in the global division of labour on the domestic labour market, have had the effect of greatly increasing social and material inequality, of increasing the numbers living on or near the margins of poverty, and of threatening many other people with partial or complete exclusion. Although not as yet widely used in the UK the term the 'New Poor' has been coined within the European Union to emphasise the consequences of some of the these changes and to identify their victims (Room 1990).

Large-scale and long-term unemployment has become an established feature of life in the present-day UK, undermining both living standards and individual self-confidence and morale. This has been especially true for male full-time workers in manufacturing industry, where there have been widespread redundancies among both blue-collar and managerial and administrative staffs. Where employment opportunities have grown, they have often been in female part-time jobs, or short-term and temporary contracts of employment. These trends have complicated the discussion of poverty in a number of ways that have still to be fully explored and intellectually absorbed. First, it is no longer true that most poverty is to be found only among those groups who are outside the labour market, those too old or too ill to work, or those unable to find work. Now many poor people are to found in the growing low-wage and under-employed sectors of the economy. Many of the social and behavioural characteristics of casual labour, first documented by Charles Booth more than a century ago, are being rediscovered (Booth 1903). Second, many of those who are still in full-time and adequately paid employment, and who cannot be described as cash-poor, nonetheless feel a profound sense of personal insecurity. This is especially true of many skilled workers in both manufacturing and the service industries, including those in clerical, administrative and managerial positions. These groups, the backbone of the middle class, have, for a very long time, been accustomed to secure, full-time, adequately rewarded employment. This has been the foundation of their sense of personal and family security. It is also the foundation upon which such long-term financial arrangements as house-mortgages and pension schemes have been predicated. But labour market rationalisation and corporate down-sizing have affected the work-force at all levels of skill and responsibility and in all regions. This has been a profound cultural shock even to those not directly affected. Thatcher wanted a society in which everyone felt themselves to be middle-class, and behaved accordingly. In fact she has proletarianised many of her own most devoted supporters, who now experience and fear institutionalised social insecurity. In France the word *precarite* captures this phenomenon: a state of precariousness in which even the most established, secure, apparently invulnerable individuals may find their circumstances suddenly and, for them, calamitously changed. This has introduced an important new social tension, which must be incorporated into the debate about poverty.

HOW IS POVERTY MEASURED?

As we have seen, the 'rediscovery' of poverty in the 1960s was based upon a measure determined by the levels of means-tested social assistance. The levels of benefit were taken as an implicit poverty line. Thus, the poor were those with household incomes that approximated to their benefit entitlement. This is a very crude measure, the more so as the basis upon which benefit levels are set has never been clearly explained, and there have been a number of important research studies which have suggested that they are clearly too low to meet all the reasonable needs of claimants (Piachaud 1979: Bradshaw 1993). However it is a starting-point and one that has been used a great deal in the academic and research environment. During the 1980s the Department of Health and Social Security (as it then was) produced the Low Income Families (LIF) statistics that used a very similar measure (UK, DHSS 1988). These statistics were based on the annual Family Expenditure Survey (FES), and took as the unit of measurement the 'benefit assessment unit' that is to say the household formation used for calculating entitlement for means-tested benefit. This approach revealed the numbers of people living in families with incomes *below* their social assistance entitlement, those *at* the benefit level, and those on the *margins* of poverty with household incomes no more than 140 per cent of the benefit-level for a household of that kind. Year-on-year calculations built up a useful picture of poverty trends over time. Disturbingly, they showed a remorseless increase throughout the 1980s in the numbers and proportion of the population in poverty, an increase which could not be explained away by increases in the real value of the benefit scale-rates which would have the effect of raising the poverty threshold.

In 1988, however, the Department discontinued this measure and replaced it with another, the Households Below Average Income (HBAI) statistics. In the HBAI, households are ranked, not in relation to their possible benefit entitlement but with respect to the mean average household income (UK, DSS 1995). Once again there is no officially recognised poverty line, but the threshold accepted most widely as a proxy for poverty is 50 per cent or less of average income after allowing for housing costs. As most countries of the European Union carry out regular surveys of family expenditure, the HBAI measure is now widely used throughout the European Union for comparative analysis, and half the average household income is usually taken as a proxy for poverty.

Both the LIF series and the HBAI statistics can be criticised. First, they both rely heavily on Family Expenditure Survey (FES) data, and so reflect any shortcomings in that data. There may for example be problems of sampling-error or non-response that distort the results. The FES only includes people who are living as members of a household. Thus whole categories of people who are very likely to be relatively poor (such as the homeless or those in institutional settings such as residential homes for the elderly) are excluded. The FES is an annual snapshot and so nothing can be learned about whether the same people are in poverty from one year to another (constituting a stubborn hard-core of poor people), or whether, although the aggregate incidence remains the same, different people drift in and out of poverty.

An additional anomaly with the LIF series was that it used the levels of means-tested social assistance as a proxy for poverty, whereas it could be argued that these levels are set precisely to lift people out of poverty. This was the principal reason why the LIF series was discontinued. But is the HBAI series an improvement? A number of particular criticisms can be singled out for comment. First, it adopts the household, rather than the benefit assessment unit or the nuclear family as the unit of measurement. But households can take many forms and may include people in a very wide range of relationships; a household can easily comprise more than one benefit assessment unit (for example where grown-up children continue to live with their parents, or where several friends are sharing accommodation). Second, it then assumes that household income is shared equally between all the members of the household. This means that any possible intra-household inequalities are over-looked. But there is abundant evidence that even within nuclear families resources may be unequally distributed, and this becomes even more likely in larger and more complex households. This is a real objection but not one that can be easily remedied. The only alternative would be to assume that all income is retained by whoever in the household earns it, that is to say that there is no sharing at all. This would clearly produce a different outcome, but only by exchanging one distortion for another, possibly even greater one. Third, concerns have been expressed about the equivalence scales that were applied to the data to allow for differences in household size. The scales used to calculate the HBAI were different from the ones used to calculate the LIF, specifically a lower weighting was given to children. This has the effect of reducing the numbers recorded as being in poverty. Certainly the use of different equivalence scales could make a significant difference to the outcome. Finally, what is being measured? Strictly speaking, the HBAI is measuring aspects of inequality of incomes, which is undoubtedly an important matter, but it is not necessarily the same as poverty.

The conclusion that must be reached is that there is no straightforward and simple measure to estimate the extent of poverty. There are, however, a range of useful statistical indicators that provide a basis for an intelligent discussion among those with the taste for it.

HOW MANY POOR ARE THERE, AND WHO ARE THEY?

The pressure group the Child Poverty Action Group has published the most detailed accessible analysis of both the LIF and the HBAI (Oppenheim and Harker 1996). The most recent statistics which have been analysed in depth using both the LIF and the HBAI measures refer to the years 1992–3 (UK, Social Services Committee 1995; UK, DSS 1995). It is useful to refer to both measures and to compare one with another, because although they differ in detail, the main thrust of the evidence from each is very clear. First of all they show that poverty in the UK is widespread. The LIF estimates that 13.7 million people were in poverty in 1992 compared with the HBAI estimate of 14.1 million. These estimates represent 25 per cent of the population. Both measures also indicate that there has been a sharp increase in the numbers and proportion in poverty since 1979. The LIF shows the increase to be from 14 per cent to 24 per cent, while the HBAI shows a sharper rise from 9 per cent of the population to 25 per cent.

Another feature of these estimates is the light they throw on the greater income inequality that has characterised the UK in the period since 1979. In the spring of 1995 the Joseph Rowntree Foundation published the findings of an exhaustive research programme into Income and Wealth (Joseph Rowntree Foundation 1994). Using the HBAI statistics, published by the Department of Social Security in 1994, the Rowntree Inquiry showed that while, during the period 1979 to 1991–2, average income (after housing costs) for the whole population grew by 33 per cent, for the lower seven-tenths of the population income growth was below that average, and for the poorest 10 per cent real income (after housing costs) may actually have fallen by between 9 and 17 per cent. This steadily growing income inequality means that the benefits of economic growth are enjoyed overwhelmingly by the already better-off sections of the community, and that the proportion of the population below the HBAI poverty threshold has grown from a low point of 7 per cent in 1972 to about 24 per cent in the early 1990s.

The statistics also give a clear indication of the social groups who are most at risk of poverty, and suggest that the social processes that put people at risk have been gradually changing so the social composition of the poor has altered. A study of the types of individuals and households most likely to experience poverty, and an examination of the circumstances that have pushed them into poverty, gives a clear indication of the underlying patterns of social change that have put some individuals and households at especial risk.

The initial, and most important, is the link between children and poverty. More than half of the total of poor people, 7.5 million people, live in households with dependent children. Indeed, the HBAI series suggest that more than half of this group, 4.3 million people, are children. This is no less than one-in-three children. The equivalent LIF figures are even bigger, 4.5 million children, or 35 per cent of the child population. Poverty has always borne heavily on children and in each year since 1979 for which we have data the proportion of the child population living in poverty has exceeded their proportion of the total population. Child poverty has increased from 10 per cent of the child population in 1979 to 33 per cent in 1992–3.

Children in poverty

There is one group of children who are particularly at risk of poverty; they live as members of a single-parent family. Of all the family types it is lone parent families who are most likely to be in poverty. They are more than twice as likely to be poor than are couples with children, and are likely to be trapped in poverty for a much longer period of time. It is clear that in recent years the traditional cultural stigma associated with family breakdown and divorce has been considerably eroded. Assumptions about the permanency of marriage have been challenged, with a somewhat more tolerant attitude towards less conventional relationships emerging. The hopes and expectations that people impose on their relationships have also begun to change. This has led to a considerable increase in family breakdown and separation. One of the consequences of this has been that an ever-growing number of women find themselves with custody of, and responsibility for, dependent children without either the financial or the emotional support of a partner. More than 75 per cent of all children in single-parent households are living in poverty, compared with fewer than 20 per cent of children living in a two-parent family.

In some instances of course, new relationships are, in due course, established and new households formed which may carry both mother and children out of poverty, but in many others this does not happen. Thus the hardship experienced by both mothers and children may be prolonged for years, possibly throughout the child's period of dependency. The dilemma for lone parents is that they have the sole responsibility for the daily care of their children, and at the same time an urgent need for income to meet the daily costs of family life. But many people find it impossible to reconcile child-care responsibilities with the parallel demands on time and energy that are entailed in holding down a job, the more so if it is a permanent, full-time job. Even if such a job can be found, the costs of buying in the necessary child-care may be excessive, so the choice is either to be poor although at work, or to be poor on social assistance. For most, the latter is the only realistic choice to be made, although to do so is to be condemned to long-term and demoralising impoverishment.

The unemployed in poverty

Unemployment has always been a major cause of poverty, and the risk of poverty is, not surprisingly, closely related to unemployment and under-employment. Unemployment has been at a very high level throughout the 1980s and into the 1990s. Accurate data on unemployment are surprisingly hard to obtain, the more so as the ways of counting the unemployed for official purposes have been frequently changed. The effect of these modifications is, however, consistent in that each change manages to produce a lower total figure than the one before. What is certain is that the official figure, at the end of 1996, of about two million is more than twice what it was in 1979, and is certainly an underestimate, and probably a substantial underestimate. The true figure is probably closer to three million people. For all these people and the families they are responsible for, the risk of poverty is real and ever-present. The HBAI data shows that three-quarters of all households where the head of household is unemployed are poor and that one-third of families dependent upon part-time earnings are poor. In more than 20 per cent of all households with incomes below the HBAI poverty threshold, the head of the household or spouse are unemployed.

The UK labour market has become increasingly volatile. Corporate down-sizing and the emergence of so-called 'flexible' labour markets are reducing the number of full-time and permanent jobs, quality jobs, in favour of part-time employment and temporary contracts. This has greatly increased the likelihood of both unemployment and under-employment and has intensified a downward pressure on wage levels which has in all likelihood increased the incidence of the working poor. The UK does not have a legally-enforceable minimum wage. Indeed, the Wages Councils which existed for many years to try and ensure minimum wages in those trades and industries characterised by low pay, have been abolished. Poverty in families on low pay cannot be ignored, and is more likely to occur where there are one or more dependent children. The HBAI data suggests that 6 per cent of children who live in families with one or more parent in full-time work, and who are either only children or have no more than one sibling, are poor. This figure rises to 20 per cent of working families with three or more children.

Poverty in older age

While it is clear that much poverty in the 1990s is closely related to conditions in the labour market, to family size and to family type, is there still a problem of poverty in older age? Certainly a great many elderly people are still poor, but their contribution to the poverty profile has diminished as the numbers of other groups in poverty have increased. Moreover the proportion of elderly people who find themselves in poverty has dropped. This drop may be attributed in large measure to the steady post-war growth in the provision of occupational pensions as part of the employment contracts of an increasing number of workers. As these contracts mature, so the numbers of people who receive an occupational pension have increased. For a steadily growing fraction of the retired population, their incomes now typically include a state pension, supplemented by an occupational pension, plus any other savings or assets they may have accumulated in earlier life. Occupational pensions vary considerably in the benefits provided. For many the value of the occupational pension will be relatively modest, but it may be suffi-cient to lift them out of poverty, even if only by a narrow margin. Thus the situation is gradually evolving of an older population divided into two broad groups. One group comprises those older people who still have to rely on the state pension, supplemented by public assistance, as their major source of support. These people continue to face a high risk of poverty. The second group contains those with more than one pension, many of whom may still hover uncomfortably on the margins of poverty, while others, particularly those from professional or senior managerial backgrounds can main-tain a comfortable, even wealthy, standard of living.

POVERTY AND SOCIAL POLICY

It is clear that a study of the debate that has taken place within the UK about the conceptualisation and definition of poverty has confused and confusing ideological roots. There is a tangle of ideas involving differing views on the relative rights and duties of the citizen and of the state, on family obligations, on the work ethic and the operation of the labour-market. Many of the same currents and cross-currents can be found in the discussions on social policy dealing with poverty. The truth is that there is not a coherent and consistent anti-poverty policy in the UK, nor is one likely to emerge in the foreseeable future.

Historically, the closest approximation to a clear set of policy ideas and administrative practices is in the thinking underlying the Victorian Poor Law. Indeed, some aspects of that conceptualisation of poverty, its causation and its cures, continue to throw a heavy shadow over the contemporary debate. In essence the Poor Law was, at least for able-bodied adults, a labour-market policy. Able-bodied adults were expected to earn their maintenance through the wages they earned from their employment. If they were unwilling to seek or accept work on the open labour market, then they, and their dependants, would be maintained in the institutional setting of a local workhouse, in conditions that were orderly and regulated, but were intended to be stigmatising to the inmate and a deterrent to others.

An important part of the story of twentieth century social policy in the UK has been the attempt to find alternative and more acceptable ways of meeting need for one group after another, without in the process undermining the discipline of the labour market as far as the great mass of able-bodied adults is concerned. To this day there remains an inescapable tension between seeking means of bringing relief to the disadvantaged without creating moral hazards and perverse incentives that are believed to undermine the work-ethic, the spirit of self-help and independence, and the rigours of the labour-market.

The role of social security

William Beveridge (1942) hoped that his ideas would provide a complete and acceptable alternative to the traditions of the Poor Law. He recommended the development of a social security system, based upon social insurance, to which everyone would belong; the payment of regular National Insurance contributions, deducted at source from wages, would earn an entitlement to a range of benefits without the need for stigmatising and administratively costly tests of individual need, merit or means. The deterrent principles of the Poor Law would be replaced by rights of citizenship, earned through membership of, and contribution to, the state system of social security.

The social security system that has developed since the 1940s includes income-replacement measures, some long-term, (such as pensions for the elderly), others with short-term interruptions in earning power, (because of, for example, sickness or temporary unemployment). It also includes income-enhancement measures, such as family credit (which supplements the wages of those with family responsibilities but with very low earnings), and child benefit (paid to all mothers with dependent children). There is also a range of other contingency benefits paid to those with identified special needs, such as disabled people. The very existence of this system has given millions of people a modicum of income security.

It has clearly helped to prevent large-scale destitution, and it has liberated people from the most extreme forms of poverty.

But Beveridge's hopes for a social security system based upon comprehensive social insurance have never been fully achieved. Parallel with the system of National Insurance there remains a large (and growing) programme of social assistance, entitlement to which is triggered not by contribution but by presumed need determined by means-testing. Moreover, there is considerable overlap between the two systems, so that for example, many elderly people who receive a state pension through the contributory National Insurance system also need to claim means-tested social assistance to raise their living standard to the publicly accepted minimum level. Similarly unemployed people quickly exhaust their entitlement to contributory unemployment benefit, and are then driven to claim means-tested assistance instead. In both cases, contributory or means-tested, the rhetoric of rights and entitlements is used, but there is no doubt that means-tested benefits are perceived by many to be stigmatising. Social assistance programmes in the UK culture carry with them a persistent and a lingering whiff of the Victorian Poor Law notion of less-eligibility and of the undeserving, which is at war with more positive ideas about citizenship and entitlement.

Nonetheless, the development of a national social security system to replace the Poor Law has been a major policy achievement of the twentieth century. But it has not been an entirely successful project. The impact of poverty upon individuals and families may have been somewhat reduced but, as we have already seen at some length, poverty has been neither abolished nor prevented. Why not? This is a complicated question, but some elements of an answer can be quickly teased out.

First, the social security system has many objectives of which reducing poverty is only one, and not necessarily the most important one. The social security system is a universal one, with coverage extended to almost everyone, rich and poor alike. There are very few people who are not directly covered by the social security system. Most people are contributors and beneficiaries for very large parts of their lives. Child benefit is paid to their mothers throughout their childhood, and they receive a retirement pension in old age. In this sense the social security scheme is universal, and no-one would suggest that it is confined or should be confined to the poor alone. What the social security system does for most people is redistribute income across their own life-cycle, raising contributions during the peak years of earning-power to enable payments to be made at other times in the life-cycle. The redistribution that takes place is horizontal rather than vertical, for it is between one age-group and another, one generation and another, or one contingency and another, rather than between richer people and poorer ones. In the modern world life-cycle adjustments of this kind are absolutely necessary, and the only matters to debate are not whether they should be done but how they are best done. It is not impossible to incorporate elements of vertical redistribution into such a social security or tax-transfer system, but it is a complication, and thus inevitably controversial. Unsurprisingly, this aspect of social security policy is not dominant (Barr and Coulter 1990).

The second reason for the continued existence of poverty is that the levels of social security benefit are clearly too low to liberate people from poverty, particularly for those who have no additional sources of income or financial support. Whether one adopts a behavioural measure such as Townsend's participation ratio, or a more formal estimate based on average household incomes, it is clear that individuals and families who are dependent on social security benefits are maintained in poverty rather than liberated from it (Townsend 1979). This situation is unlikely to change. The economic and political costs of systematically raising benefits to an acceptable level would be high, and although many people would welcome the outcome they would not welcome the means necessary to achieve the outcome. Debate on the issue would however become much clearer if the inadequacy of benefit levels could be recognised more openly. For example, it could be acknowledged that social security payments only make a contribution to a minimally acceptable living standard, they do not guarantee it. Beveridge himself would not have had too much difficulty with this idea. He was very clear that, as a matter of policy, benefit levels should be set at no more than subsistence level. They should meet basic needs and ensure survival, but they were not, and should not be, seen as maintaining a customary living standard. Social security should provide a safety net, beyond which individuals and families would supplement through savings and private provision, or from alternative charitable sources. But this aspect of Beveridge's thinking (whatever its merits) is not echoed in official pronouncements. Here the social security rhetoric asserts, unconvincingly but persistently, that benefits are sufficient to meet need, although the basis upon which such assertions have been made are not transparent. The official dilemma is that since 1934, the law governing means-tested assistance has imposed upon the social security authorities a duty to meet individual and family need. But this duty has to be realised in the real world of Treasury anxiety about the overall levels of public expenditure; intense competition for scarce public resources to finance programmes that all command widespread public support (such as health care, education, housing and so on); a public desire for improved services but a distaste for the taxation regimes that would raise the revenues needed; an increasingly volatile labour-market; long-term demographic trends which will alter the ratio of earners and dependants; and changes in patterns of social life which introduce new and unpredictable sources of long-term income insecurity. In this context maintaining a fiction about the adequacy of benefits hinders rational debate.

The third reason is that many people fail to claim benefits to which they are entitled (Hill 1990: 92–110). In some cases, people may be unaware of their entitlements, and so do not claim through ignorance; in other cases there may be uncertainty about how to make a claim. But the problem of low take-up is most marked, and most persistent, with means-tested benefits, where the procedures for claiming may be long-winded and off-putting, and where the sense of stigma may be strongest. Efforts have been made to improve take-up rates, although they have only had a limited success. In some cases the government, itself, has campaigned vigorously to ensure a higher take-up rate for some benefits. Campaigns of this kind have usually been associated with the introduction of a new or radically reorganised benefit to which the authorities attach special significance. But take-up campaigns have more usually been sponsored by other public authorities. Of particular importance here has been the development of a self-conscious welfare rights perspective among many local authorities as part of an attempt to develop strong local anti-poverty policies. Work of this kind is of course useful, it marginally increases the income of some of the poorest families, it helps the social security system itself to fulfil its objectives, and it gives a higher profile to the need for coherent anti-poverty measures to be developed.

In some senses then the social security system continues to be as much part of the problem as it is part of the solution, incorporating as it does so many of the conflicting ideas and contested practices that have characterised the UK welfare debate throughout the twentieth century. Social security will, of course, continue to have a crucial part to play in the struggle to reduce poverty, but it has to be seen as only one important element in that struggle. It needs to be strongly reinforced by associated and parallel anti-poverty policy initiatives.

THE POLICY PRIORITIES

What policy priorities need to be reviewed as the century draws to a close? Here the concern should not be with the technical detail of UK social policy, not because this is unimportant, for it is absolutely vital, but because there are a number of bigger, overarching, issues that are of relevance not just to the UK but globally. Are there then issues that have universal resonance, that raise questions and dilemmas that apply everywhere? Such challenging issues must include questions relating to employment and unemployment, to the capacity for perpetual and sustainable economic growth, and to the underlying issue of wealth distribution and redistribution.

While continuing efforts must be made to make the UK social security system more responsive to need, and particularly to enable it to adapt to changing circumstances and underlying patterns of social life, an equally important task is to try to reduce as far as possible the circumstances which force people to make claims upon the social security system. Are there ways in which poverty can be prevented, rather than simply relieved? Here the single most important question to be confronted, not just for poverty prevention but for a much wider range of concerns about social integration and cohesion, is that of employment.

The goal of full employment

Most people keep themselves and their families out of poverty through working and earning. Most people want to work, not only for the money they can earn, but also because of the satisfactions they gain from shared activity, and from the social networks that work opens up. This is true even when the job itself is arduous, or where working conditions are hard, even dangerous. Indeed it is precisely in these working environments that social solidarity is most marked. For many people their own sense of worth and self-esteem is bound up with their jobs, and with the social contribution they are thus able to make, as well as with the financial rewards they may receive.

The greatest single challenge facing UK society is posed by continued high levels of unemployment and under-employment. The UK economy has, in recent years, seen a pattern of short-lived booms followed by more prolonged recessions, with unemployment levels falling and then rising again, but always settling at a level higher than that experienced at the start of the cycle. Permanent full-time jobs are replaced by short-term, temporary, or part-time ones. Similarly, a steady downward pressure on wage-levels, particularly for semi-skilled or unskilled employment, means that maintaining the living standard even for those in work is threatened.

Unemployment, and the fear of unemployment, with the associated loss of a sense of personal and social security have severe consequences for both individuals and families. The implications for social welfare programmes, and ultimately for the stability of the social order and the quality of life, are as severe. Without reasonable assurances about the availability of regular work, which is rewarded by wages and salaries paid at levels that enable people to support themselves and their families at an acceptable standard of living, then coherent long-term responsible family financial planning, ranging from mortgage arrangements for house purchase, to planned savings and controlled household budgeting habits, become hazardous if not impossible to formulate and implement. Similarly, if the labour market continues to fail on the scale that it has in recent years, then the capacity of the state to maintain stabilising programmes of income support will be fatally undermined. The long-term planning and organisation necessary to underpin pension schemes or health care programmes that can be relied upon will also be jeopardised.

A first priority for public policy must be to secure a return to fuller and more secure employment. Only in this way will the socially divisive and destructive pressures that exclusion from the labour market generates be reduced. Only in this way will the intolerable pressure on public finance to underwrite the continuing and growing costs of unemployment be alleviated. Only in this way will the tax-base be restored so that other valuable social programmes can be funded. Only in this way will the potential productivity and wealth creation locked up in an army of unemployed people be released.

Although higher levels of employment, paid at wage rates that will keep individuals and families out of poverty, are clearly matters of great public importance, are they matters that government intervention can help to achieve? Apologists for a free-market approach to public policy insist that they are not. The market must be allowed to prevail, and if so allowed will achieve the best attainable outcome. Globalisation and flexible labour markets may be uncomfortable for some, but, it is argued, any attempt to regulate the labour market will fail. For the Conservative governments during the 1980s and early 1990s removing perceived obstacles to a flexible labour market was a high priority, involving a determined legislative attack on the trade-union movement, and a constant stream of modifications to the social security regulations, many of which discriminated against the unemployed and undermined their capacity to resist the new labour-market pressures. For the same reason, the government has opposed, and resisted, all attempts within the European Union to establish a social chapter which sets certain minimum standards within the labour market. These have been presented as actually damaging to national economies, leading to a loss of jobs rather than their creation. From this perspective, it is long-term economic growth alone that will create jobs and wealth, and thanks to the 'trickle-down' effect even the poorest in the community will benefit from greater national wealth. However, the evidence on this matter is not encouraging. The years of Conservative government since 1979 have seen the UK economy grow, albeit fitfully and unevenly, but the trickle-down effect has not worked to any significant extent. On the contrary, as the Rowntree Inquiry revealed, inequality has greatly increased and the most deprived groups in the community have shared little, if at all, in the benefits of rising national prosperity. The mantra of the unregulated free market may act as little more than an ideological cover for sectional advantage and, at the extreme, of unbridled corporate greed.

The prospects for economic growth

It is certainly true that a dynamic and expanding economy makes it easier to increase individual rewards, and will create the wealth upon which social policies and programmes depend. So, for those with a serious concern about poverty, the debate certainly involves the case for growth. But it also involves a concern for the ways in which that wealth is distributed and redistributed. As far as economic growth itself is concerned the UK debate is influenced by two major concerns: that growth alone will neither be sufficient, nor environmentally sustainable. Is it the case that economic recovery and growth will lead to a return towards fuller employment? The prospect of economic growth occurring without creating jobs becomes more pressing. Suppose that the labour market of the future remains one where job insecurity is widespread and permanent, where long-term planning is impossible or foolhardy, where large numbers of people are wholly excluded from the world of work and remain dependent upon increasingly-stretched public services for their every need. The fear that this may be the pattern for the future, scarred by a partial but serious and ineradicable market failure, has contributed to a more widespread discussion in some circles about more radical approaches to the distribution of income, such as the payment of a universal basic citizen's income for all, irrespective of their employment. Likewise the argument that it is impossible or undesirable to try to impose a minimum wage, has raised the question about whether it might be more fruitful to talk about establishing not a minimum, but a maximum wage, only to be exceeded with careful and full public justification.

The prospects for the environment

Meanwhile fears about the prospects for sustainable growth have been powerfully fuelled by the evidence and arguments of the environmentalists. Issues of resource depletion, widespread pollution and degradation of natural resources, the dangers of global warming and so on, have raised serious questions about the sustainability of economic growth driven by ever-increasing personal consumption.

It is hard to see that the free market is able to offer a sensible solution to either of these concerns, other than to urge blind optimism, or simple faith, in its superiority: an optimism that is confounded by the evidence, and a faith that is undermined by experience.

Another approach is to look to sensible regulation of the market. What the market does well, it should be encouraged to do, but where it fails in ways that cannot simply be ignored, then regulation or some other form of public intervention is required. Markets respond more powerfully to private demands because they can be immediately expressed, than to collective demands, which have to be collectively articulated through a political mechanism.

The dynamic individualism of the market needs the counterweight of recognised social goals and ambitions that can only be

achieved collectively. These start with the need for global survival
and the protection of the global environment, a goal that is
certainly on a par with widely recognised and publicly-financed
needs for national defence. Can environmentally sustainable
economic growth be achieved in ways that do not enrich one corner
of the globe at the expense of the rest? Fundamentally, the same
processes that cause the impoverishment of vulnerable groups
within a country, contribute to gross inequalities between countries
and regions of the world. Can global economic growth be achieved
that is both sustainable and equitable?

The prospects for the redistribution of wealth

If it is clear that the unregulated operation of the market leads *inter
alia* to intolerable inequalities that, for the victims, are positively
harmful, even life-threatening, and for everyone are socially disfig-
uring and ultimately destructive, then consideration must be given
to finding more effective ways to reduce poverty and inequality.
Internationally, this will require economic and trading relationships
that are not one-sided, but that bring benefits to all. This means
international co-operation to reduce the risks of war between
nations, and long-term strategic international collaboration to
attack epidemic disease, and to enhance the living standards and
quality of life of the most impoverished populations of the world.

Nationally there needs to be serious discussion of both the
creation and the distribution of wealth and well-being. Currently
unfashionable themes, such as wages and income policy, must be
reconsidered, even if only to be rejected as undesirable or unwork-
able, as must a coherent taxation policy. The aim must be to enable
the largest number of people to become self-supporting through
their own adequately paid work, with protection for those too
young, too old or too ill to hold down jobs. In the UK at the
moment there is no coherent public discussion on any of these
matters. On the contrary, both taxation policy and the case for
redistribution appear to be politically taboo subjects, upon which
even the Labour Party is dismayingly quiet. But this reticence
cannot last for ever.

CONCLUSION

As the social crisis in the UK grows more intense, as social insecurity and uncertainty become ever more widespread and corrosive, as the miracles of the free market continue to be promised for tomorrow but never achieved today, so attention will once again be focused on the major social challenges so eloquently and tragically expressed in persistent poverty, at the local, national and international levels. The challenge thus becomes, how to work towards a national and a world order in which everyone has the capacity to make informed choices about their own lives, and the opportunity to realise their potential, thereby fulfilling themselves in ways that, as though guided by an invisible hand, enrich and strengthen the social bonds that unite and dignify us all.

REFERENCES

Abel-Smith, B, and Townsend, P. (1965) *The Poor and the Poorest* London: Bell.

Barr, N. and Coulter, F. (1990) 'Social Security: Solution or Problem', in Hills, J. (ed.) *The State of Welfare*, Oxford: Clarendon Press.

Beveridge, W. (1942) *Social Insurance and Allied Services* (CMND 6404), London: HMSO.

Booth, C. (1903) *Life and Labour of the People of London*, London: Macmillan.

Bradshaw, J. (ed.) (1993) *Household Budgets and Living Standards*, York: Joseph Rowntree Foundation.

Greve, J. (1964) *London's Homeless*, London: Bell.

Hill, M. (1990) *Social Security Policy in Britain*, Aldershot: Edward Elgar.

Joseph Rowntree Foundation (1994) *Inquiry into Income and Wealth* (Volumes 1 and 2), York: Joseph Rowntree Foundation.

Murray, C. (1984) *Losing Ground: American Social Policy 1950–80*, New York: Basic Books.

—— (1990) *The Emerging British Underclass*, London: Institute of Economic Affairs.

Oppenheim, C. and Harker, L. (1996) *Poverty: The Facts* (3rd edn), London: Child Poverty Action Group.

Piachaud, D. (1979) *The Cost of a Child* (Poverty Pamphlet 43), London: Child Poverty Action Group.

—— (1987) 'Problems in the Definition and Measurement of Poverty', *Journal of Social Policy* 16 (2): 147–64.

Room, G., Lawson, R. and Laczko, F. (1989) "New Poverty" in the European Community', *Policy and Politics* 17 (2): 165–76

Room, G. (1990) *'New Poverty' in the European Community*, London: Macmillan.

Rowntree, S. (1901) *Poverty: a Study of Town Life*, London: Macmillan.

—— (1937) *The Human Needs of Labour*, London: Longmans, Green.

—— (1941) *Poverty and Progress*, London: Longmans.

Townsend, P. (1957) *The Family Life of Old People*, London: Routledge and Kegan Paul.

—— (1979) *Poverty in the United Kingdom*, Harmondsworth: Penguin Books.

United Kingdom, Department of Health and Social Security (UK, DHSS) (1988) *Low Income Families 1985*, London: DHSS.

United Kingdom, Department of Social Security (UK, DSS) (1995) *Households Below Average Income, A Statistical Analysis 1979–1992/3*, London: HMSO.

United Kingdom, Social Services Committee (1995) *First Report: Low Income Statistics: Low Income Families (LIF) 1989–1992*, London: HMSO.

Chapter 10

United States of America

James Midgley and Michelle Livermore

The United States of America (US) is viewed by its citizens as a land of freedom and opportunity, a place where success is guaranteed to anyone who has drive and ambition. Wealth, prestige and a comfortable life style await those who have the determination to succeed. Millions of people in other countries share this belief. Indeed, during this century, America has been perceived internationally as a paragon for those who seek prosperity and wealth.

While it is true that the country has many very wealthy people, and that their opulent life styles are envied all over the world, poverty is widespread. There are currently 39 million people in America who have incomes below the government's poverty line. They comprise more than 15 per cent of the population (US, Bureau of the Census 1995). The contrast between poverty and wealth is particularly stark. In most American cities, the living standards of people in the prosperous suburbs are among the highest in the world. On the other hand, urban blight, homelessness, crime and poverty comprise a way of life for many in the inner cities. Similarly, substantial numbers of Americans in the rural areas continue to live in condition of deprivation.

This chapter examines poverty in America. It begins by providing a brief country profile and then reviews the different ways poverty has been defined. The incidence of poverty is described with reference to both historical and contemporary data. The groups most affected are also identified. Then a review of the policy responses to the poverty problem is presented. It describes income support and community-based anti-poverty programmes and examines various economic and social interventions that address the causes of poverty. In discussing policy responses to poverty, the theoretical explanations of the causes of poverty which underlay these policies and programmes are discussed. Policy responses are not implemented in a vacuum but give expression to underlying ideas about the nature and origins of the poverty problem.

PROFILE OF THE UNITED STATES

The US is a federation of 50 states located in the northern half of the western hemisphere. Covering 9,158,925 square kilometres of land, the country is sizeable by international standards (US, Bureau of the Census 1995). The total population was in excess of 260 million as of 1 July 1994 (US, Bureau of the Census 1995). According to 1992 data, 203 million Americans lived in metropolitan areas and 51 million lived in non-metropolitan areas (US, Bureau of the Census 1995). Politically, America is a democracy with a separation of powers between three branches of government. These are the executive, legislative and judicial branches. The executive and legislative branches are elected by individuals who cast votes in elections.

American history reveals much about the composition of its population. After rebelling against British colonial rule in 1776, the American colonies formed their own nation. The population was comprised mostly of individuals of European origin (notably English, French and Spanish). In addition, slavery brought many Africans to America. An open immigration policy encouraged many other Europeans to immigrate and many people of Irish, Italian, German, Chinese, Japanese and other national origins came to the country.

Known as a melting pot, the American population is quite diverse. In 1994, the country's population was made up of 192 million Caucasians (or whites), 31 million African Americans (or blacks), 26 million of Hispanic origin, 8.4 million Asians and Pacific Islanders and 1.9 million Native Americans (US, Bureau of the Census 1995). However, even those classified as Caucasian come from diverse backgrounds and include Italians, Dutch, Ukrainians, Irish, French and many others.

In addition to its ethnic diversity, the American population is ageing. Like many other industrial countries, the proportion of the population over 65 years is increasing; currently it is 12.8 per cent. This trend will continue as the 70 million Americans who are now between 40 and 64 (currently 27.2 per cent of the population) reach 65. Of the remainder, 31.3 per cent are aged between 20 and 39 years and 28.8 per cent are 19 years or under.

Social and economic indicators reveal that living conditions are very mixed. America's per capita gross national product was US$24,740 in 1995 (World Bank 1995). While the median income for men in 1993 was US$21,102, it was only US$11,046 for women. In terms of education, 81 per cent of those aged 25 and more had received a high school or university education by 1994 (US, Bureau of the Census 1995). According to the World Bank (1995), both the total literacy rate and female literacy rates in 1990 were over 95 per cent. In 1993, the infant mortality rate was nine per 1,000 live births and life expectancy at birth was 76 years (World Bank 1995).

THE DEFINITION OF POVERTY

Envisioning the poor in America brings to mind scenes of material deprivation including dirty, hungry children, dilapidated buildings and feelings of hopelessness and despair. Michael Harrington (1962) brought these scenes into the national spotlight in his book *The Other America*. However, as in other countries, American poverty is viewed differently by different people. Definitions vary between those who view poverty as an absolute condition and those who see poverty as a relative condition (Townsend 1970).

In order to make the concept of poverty more tangible, attempts have been made to devise objective measures of poverty based on income. Mollie Orshansky of the Social Security Administration developed a measure in 1963 that was accepted as the country's official poverty level (US, Department of Health, Eduation and Welfare 1976). This measure defined a poverty line of US$3,000 per year for a family of four, based on the Department of Agriculture's economy food plan of 1961. Orshansky's formula multiplied the economy food plan by three, since one third of a typical family's total household expenditures was spent on food. The intention of this poverty line was to compute the income level at which individuals could meet their basic needs. This level was then used to determine the numbers whose needs were unmet.

Although the Orshansky poverty line has been modified over the years, it continues to serve as the predominant measure of American poverty. Today, the federal government defines a range of poverty thresholds adjusted for the size of the family, the age of the householder and the number of children under 18 years of age. Poverty thresholds are updated annually and adjusted for inflation. In 1993, the poverty threshold for a family of four was US$14,763 (US, Bureau of the Census 1995).

THE INCIDENCE OF POVERTY

When examining the incidence of poverty in America, several factors need to be considered. These include overall historical poverty trends, the effects of economic recessions and the differential distribution of poverty on the basis on age, race, gender, area of residence and marital status. In addition, it must be remembered that ideological presuppositions play a major role in conceptualisations of poverty and shape the definitions which are used. Throughout American history, the definition of poverty has changed as attitudes and beliefs regarding poor people have shifted. As standards of living in the country have risen, the perception of poverty has changed. In colonial days, poverty was regarded as natural. The numerous hardships that plagued the lives of Native Americans and early frontiersmen and women during these times were to be expected and poverty was a fact of life (Rothman and Rothman 1972).

While Enlightenment ideas re-framed popular conceptions of poverty as unacceptable and capable of being eradicated, it also encouraged the view that poor people were at least partly responsible for their situation (Rothman and Rothman 1972). Behavioural factors such as a lack of ambition and willingness to work were identified as causes of poverty. In the mid-1800s, as urbanisation increased rapidly and as more migrants flocked to the country, perceptions of poverty shifted from emphasising material deprivation to a concern with the proliferation of pauperism and dependency on assistance. Pauperism is an extreme level of indigence in which dependence on public or private charity is a key factor.

The Great Depression of the 1930s fostered the view that poverty was caused by structural factors. As large numbers of Americans lost their jobs and fell into poverty, it became increasingly difficult to attribute blame to individual causes. As unemployment soared and more and more people became destitute, theories that explained poverty with reference to wider economic and social conditions gained popularity. These beliefs fostered the idea that the solution to poverty could best be found through concerted government action at the national level.

Although official poverty data have only been collected since the 1960s, general health indicators tell much about social conditions before that time. These indicators include infant mortality rates and life expectancy which reveal a gradual improvement in the well-being of Americans over the past decades. For instance, life expectancy at birth rose from 50 years in 1910 to 69.7 years in 1960. Infant mortality declined from 99.9 per 1,000 live births in 1915 to 26 per 1,000 live births in 1960 (US, Bureau of the Census 1975).

Official poverty data show fluctuations in the proportion of the population living in poverty since the 1960s. In the early 1960s, poverty rates were very high but during the 1960 and 1970s, they declined steadily until the early 1980s when a resurgence was recorded. The census data shown in Table 10.1 reveal that 22.2 per cent of the population lived below the poverty line in 1960. This figure dropped to 12.6 per cent in 1970. However, in the 1980s, poverty began to increase again. Census data for 1980 reveal that 13 per cent of the population lived below the poverty line. In 1983, the figure reached a high of 15.2 per cent. It fell to 13.5 per cent in 1990 but increased again to 14.5 per cent in 1992 and 15.1 per cent in 1993 (US, Bureau of the Census 1995).

GROUPS MOST AFFECTED BY POVERTY

Looking beyond national trends, it is clear that poverty affects some groups more that others. Differences include age, race, family structure and place of residence. Table 10.1 summarises the main features of American poverty.

Since the mid-1970s, the largest group of individuals living in poverty have been children. In 1992, 39.6 per cent of the American poor were children under 18 years of age. This equates to 21.9 per cent of all children. In contrast, before this time, the elderly (people age 65 and over) had the highest level of poverty of any age group. In 1970, 24.6 per cent of all seniors lived in poverty compared to 12.2 per cent in 1993 (US, Bureau of the Census 1995).

Race is another important aspect of America's poverty profile. Even though the majority of people who live below the poverty line in 1992 were white (66.5 per cent), most minority groups have a higher rate of poverty than whites. For instance, 33.1 per cent of African Americans and 30.6 per cent of Hispanics lived below the poverty line in 1993, while only 12.2 per cent of whites were poor

Table 10.1 Poverty in the United States

Poverty level for a household of four in 1993	US$14,763
Each group (%) living below the poverty level	
All races	15.1
White	12.2
Black	33.1
Hispanic	30.6
Children under 18	40.0
Female headed families	34.9
Male headed families	15.6
Families headed by married couples	10.0
Poverty rate (%): 1960–93	
1960	22.2
1966	14.7
1970	12.6
1983	15.2
1990	13.5
1993	15.1

Source: US, Bureau of the Census.

(US, Bureau of the Census 1995). Family structure and gender are other variables. In 1992, 34.9 per cent of female-headed families lived in poverty compared to 15.6 per cent of male-headed families and 6.2 per cent of married couples (US, Bureau of the Census 1993). Poverty is also related to location. As most of America's population has congregated in the cities, so have the poor. By 1992, 74.2 per cent of poor people lived in metropolitan areas (US, Bureau of the Census 1993).

In addition, the degree of poverty and its duration also varies. Segalman and Asoke (1981) have identified three types of impoverished groups who experience different degrees of poverty for different periods of time. The transitional poor experience poverty for only a relatively short period of time. They become poor because of unemployment, family break-up and other factors which exert only a temporary effect on their status. The marginal poor contain the long-term working poor and are comprised of those who have low incomes but who manage to stay just above or on the poverty line. Finally, the residual poor are those who remain in poverty for an extended period of time. They are often dependent on government assistance and are often identified as the 'underclass' (Wilson 1987).

POLICY RESPONSES TO THE POVERTY PROBLEM

Policy responses to the poverty problem are not formulated in a vacuum but mirror wider beliefs about the nature and causes of poverty. These beliefs not only arise out of popular views about poverty but reflect the ideas of American social scientists who have achieved international recognition for their work in the field. Their ideas have formed the basis for many American policy interventions.

Some explanations of the causes of poverty emphasise factors which operate at the individual level. Others stress the role of wider social and economic factors. The former theories attribute poverty to personal inadequacy, stressing the role of irresponsibility and low levels of ambition. These explanations contend that poverty is due to the inability of individuals to exploit the opportunities afforded by America's dynamic economy and open social system. Some of these theories go deeper claiming that personal inadequacy is caused by low intelligence (Murray and Herrnstein 1994), negative cultural values (Lewis 1966), a low motivation to work (Mead 1986, 1996) and low levels of education (Becker 1964; Schultz 1960, 1981).

Theories that stress the role of social and economic factors in the aetiology of poverty include explanations that attribute poverty to the American class system and the way it inhibits upward mobility (Bowles and Gintis 1976; Merton 1957). Another emphasises declining opportunities for remunerative employment caused by de-industrialisation and economic decline in inner city areas (Bluestone and Harrison 1982; Wilson 1987). Some explanations even blame government social programmes which allegedly deter people from working and make them dependent on the state (Murray 1984). These theories emphasise causative factors over which individuals have little control and they imply that solutions to the poverty problem must be found through policies implemented at the national level.

These disparate approaches to explaining poverty are reflected in the many policies and programmes which have been introduced over the years. In most cases, theoretical explanations of the causes of poverty are implicit in the policies adopted by government, but in some cases, policy interventions have been explicitly based on social science ideas.

Although a great variety of charitable and non-formal activities contribute to the amelioration of poverty in American society, the following discussion of policy responses to the poverty problem will focus largely on government programmes. However, it must be recognised that the American government has long supported a pluralistic approach to poverty alleviation in which the activities of voluntary organisations, and even commercial human service enterprises are not only recognised and encouraged but funded.

Income-support programmes

As in other societies, non-formal welfare institutions operating through the family, community and church have been extensively utilised by needy American people. Long before colonisation, the indigenous population had well developed institutions of this kind which catered for orphans, the elderly and others in need. Similar practices existed among the settlers but here, traditional forms of support were supplemented by formal charitable organisations managed by both religious and secular bodies. During the nineteenth century, these activities evolved into a complex system of philanthropic relief. Most large American cities had extensive systems of support which catered for the destitute and other needy groups (Leiby 1978).

It was widely accepted in the nineteenth century that poverty was the result of either individual inadequacy or misfortune. Reflecting this individualist interpretation, a sharp distinction was drawn between the deserving and undeserving poor. The former group, which comprised widows, needy children, the destitute elderly and disabled were believed to be poor through no fault of their own. It was generally agreed that they were deserving of charitable help. On the other hand, the latter group were believed to be poor because of insobriety, irresponsibility and indolence. Since this group had chosen to live a dissolute life, they were not only denied charitable assistance but were regarded as a 'dangerous class' who should be controlled and compelled to work. This distinction between the deserving and undeserving poor has proved to be surprisingly durable and continues to pervade policy thinking today.

In addition to the welfare services provided by the charities, the government also intervened to deal with poverty. Many American colonies enacted poor law legislation based directly on the Elizabethan statute of 1601. During the nineteenth century, however, many followed the British practice of incarcerating applicants for poor relief in residential facilities. This development reflected the increasingly punitive attitudes of many middle- and upper-class people towards the poor and especially the able-bodied, undeserving poor. The adoption of these punitive approaches also reflected a popular dislike for government intervention. It was widely accepted that the charities rather than government should assist those in need (Leiby 1978).

Nevertheless, towards the end of the nineteenth century, government services designed to reduce and even prevent poverty gradually expanded. In addition to general relief provided through the Poor Laws, many states introduced means-tested mothers' pensions to assist widows with children. In some states, these programmes also permitted payments to women who had been deserted by their husbands (Skocpol 1992). These programmes were later enhanced by the introduction of old age assistance and workmen's compensation both of which were designed to help people who could no longer earn their livelihood through regular employment. Workmen's compensation expanded rapidly in the early decades of this century and by 1920, 42 states had established programmes of this kind (Day 1989). Old age assistance programmes were not as widely adopted and only 11 states had programmes of this kind by the end of the 1920s (Day 1989).

The Great Depression persuaded many that the voluntary organisations and states were not capable of effectively addressing the poverty problem. During the 1930s, President Roosevelt's administration introduced, as a part of the New Deal, a variety of programmes which, it was hoped, would eradicate poverty. The New Deal was based on the assumption that government economic policies inspired by Keynesian ideas would promote steady growth and ensure full employment. Policy makers believed that employment in an ever expanding economy would be the primary means for abolishing poverty in American society (Patterson 1994).

Income-support programmes were also introduced, as a part of the New Deal, to cater to those who could not work or who were temporarily unemployed. These groups included the unemployed and those who were out of work because of illness or a work-related injury. Since the elderly and disabled could not be expected to work, they were entitled to receive indefinite income support. Widows and deserted women were also assisted. Most of these provisions were introduced in terms of the 1935 Social Security Act but others, such as disability insurance were added in later amendments. Sixty years later, the Social Security Act continues to provide statutory authority for a variety of American income-support programmes (Kingson and Berkowitz 1993).

Although the Social Security Act is widely regarded as a major historical step in the evolution of the American welfare state, it did not include a health-care programme and in this respect, American social policy differs significantly from that of most other developed nations. In the mid-1960s, the addition of health care insurance for the elderly (Medicare), and a means-tested health-care programme for the indigent (Medicaid), broadened the scope of American welfarism but neither provided the same level of coverage as in other advanced welfare states. On the other hand, the War on Poverty programmes introduced as a part of President Johnson's Great Society initiative at this time, have lead the world in locality-based anti-poverty strategies.

The retirement, survivors and disability provisions of the Social Security Act form the core and the largest component of the country's income-support programme. In the United States, these insurance programmes are known as social security. Social security is administered by the federal government's Social Security Administration through 1,250 regional offices. It currently pays benefits to some 33 million elderly people and more than three million disabled people at an annual cost of almost US$300 billion per year (Kingson and Berkowitz 1993). Although the programme has enjoyed wide public support, it has recently received increasing media attention because of doubts about its long-term fiscal viability.

The means-tested elements of the federal government's income-support programme has become controversial. Known as Aid to Families with Dependent Children (AFDC) or colloquially as 'welfare', it was intended to assist families with children whose incomes had been interrupted or terminated through the death, illness or desertion of the breadwinner. The programme was intended to serve as a supplementary safety net to the social insurance component of the Social Security Act, but, over the years, the numbers receiving AFDC has increased significantly. Currently, some 14 million persons receive AFDC at a cost of about US$25 billion (Abramovitz 1995). In addition, they receive food vouchers and medical care and many are eligible for housing and education assistance as well.

Recent developments in social assistance have reinforced the view that poverty is caused by individual factors and particularly by low levels of education, poor work habits and negative social values, all of which are inimical to mainstream American beliefs about ambition, hard work and individual effort. The ideas of writers such as Murray (1984) and Mead (1986, 1996) have been particularly influential in shaping the new policy approaches which have emerged in income-support policy. Mead's insistence that the poor are disinterested in utilising the country's abundant employment opportunities has formed the basis for the 'work-fare' policies which now characterise social assistance in many states.

These ideas are consonant with the changes introduced over the last 15 years. During the Reagan Presidency in the 1980s, various budgetary and other restrictions were imposed and, with the enactment of the 1988 Family Support Act, new eligibility requirements were introduced. The AFDC programme is currently undergoing major changes. The federal government has permitted states to introduce many more eligibility requirements and with the enactment of the Personal Responsibility and Work Opportunity Reconciliation Act of 1996, a substantial measure of decentralisation has been introduced. This legislation will permit greater flexibility in the way the states use federal resources to administer income assistance programmes.

Community-based anti-poverty programmes

Communitarian ideas have long exerted a powerful influence in American culture (Etzioni 1993). While individualism is a dominant ideology, Americans also believe strongly in the virtues of local, neighbourhood self-help. These ideas have influenced community-based programmes which emphasise the role of local participation in addressing social needs. Proponents of this approach believe that poverty can best be addressed at the community level by involving local people in a variety of social, political and economic activities that raise incomes and enhance the quality-of-life.

America has been a pioneer of locality-based anti-poverty programmes directed at deprived, low income communities. The most comprehensive attempt to attack poverty through community-based interventions was President Johnson's War on Poverty of the mid-1960s. The Economic Opportunity Act created a variety of programmes including Operation Head Start, the volunteer (VISTA) programme, the Job Corps and the Upward Bound Program but its key component was the Community Action Program which created local community action agencies in low income areas to ensure the 'maximum feasible participation' of the poor in local anti-poverty initiatives. However, this programme was never fully funded and when it became associated with the civil rights movement, its political support dwindled. Nevertheless, as Quadagno (1994) has shown, the Community Action Program played a major role in enfranchising African Americans and securing a base for their political activities.

Community-based anti-poverty programmes continue to have appeal in America but there have been few systematic attempts to evaluate their effectiveness. Many have mobilised low income people for political activities and their role in 'empowering' the poor is frequently emphasised in the literature (Mondros and Wilson 1994; Simon 1994). On the other hand, some experts believe that more emphasis on local economic development is needed. They believe that programmes which stimulate local enterprises and create jobs are most likely to reduce poverty (Blakely 1994; Galaway and Hudson 1994; Halpern 1995).

The need for local economic development is currently receiving more attention in policy circles. The Clinton administration's community-based enterprise zones which cater for both urban and rural communities gives expression to these ideas. Based on a British concept, enterprise zones offer attractive investment incentives and reduce regulation in an attempt to attract businesses. Although the Bush administration and several states had previously promoted the approach, it has been during the Clinton administration that it has been vigorously promoted (Blakely 1994).

National economic and social development programmes

The dominance of means-tested programmes, such as AFDC, in American anti-poverty programmes fosters the belief that the poor are comprised of a core of unemployed people who are dependent on governmental aid. These programmes obscure the fact that there are millions of poor people who work every day but whose incomes are too low to provide an adequate standard of living. In 1992, 40.3 per cent of poor people aged 16 years and over worked regularly (US, Bureau of the Census 1993). For these people, better paying jobs are widely regarded as the solution to the problem. However, there is a good deal of evidence to show that incomes have stagnated during the last 20 years (Danziger and Gottschalk 1995; Reich 1991). While rapid economic growth in the decades following the Second World War raised the incomes of many millions of Americans, economic growth since the 1970s has been sluggish. The creation of well-paying employment opportunities poses a major challenge and requires policy approaches which differ significantly from traditional welfare responses. Many experts believe that large-scale anti-poverty interventions that affect a variety of economic, educational and other determinants of poverty are urgently needed.

In addition, there is recognition that specific measures which ensure adequate minimum incomes for those who work are needed. These include minimum wage policies and the use of the earned income-tax credit. America has long implemented a minimum wage policy. Currently, employers are mandated to pay a minimum wage of US$4.75 which will increase to US$5.15 in July 1997. The earned income-tax credit, which is designed to help low income workers by providing tax refunds, was introduced in 1975 and has since been expanded significantly. In 1993, the maximum tax credit payable was 19.5 per cent of income and about 14 million Americans families benefited from the programme. Under legislation introduced in 1993, an additional 4.7 million families have been added to the programme. The total cost of the programme is about US$25 billion which is about the same amount spent on the AFDC programme each year (Danziger and Gottschalk 1995).

The earned-income tax credit is an effective way of raising the incomes of the working poor. However, writers such as Wilson (1987) believe that the problem of low incomes will only be resolved when the economy expands and creates well-paying, secure jobs. He argues that poverty is inextricably linked to the economic changes which have taken place over the last two decades. De-industrialisation has had a particularly damaging impact on standards of living in inner city areas. Industries which previously employed many semi- and low-skilled blue-collar workers have closed with the result that unemployment in inner city areas has

242 James Midgley and Michelle Livermore

increased. Because of a mismatch between people's skills and employment opportunities, whole communities have sunk into poverty. The absence of transport services which can take local people to the suburbs in search of employment further increases their isolation. To make matters worse, crime, violence and drug use has increased. The result is the emergence of an underclass of deprived people whose prospects are bleak. While some children in the inner city will secure educational qualifications which will equip them for remunerative employment, most will grow up with little hope. Among them, many males will become involved in criminal activities and spend a good part of their lives in prison. Those who acquire educational qualifications and find employment are likely to leave the inner city and move to the suburbs. Because of the absence of successful role models for other children and young people, the problem is perpetuated. In addition, some writers such as Massey and Denton (1993) believe that the problem is exacerbated by racial antagonisms. They argue that racism is a major reason for the increasing segregation of ethnic minorities in inner city ghetto areas.

Policy responses emerging out of the view that poverty is caused by economic decline and de-industrialisation stress the use of macroeconomic policy interventions to promote investment, stimulate consumer demand, raise productivity, foster exports and implement other measures which will increase economic growth. Some economists believe that stagnating incomes and persistent poverty are due to sluggish growth and particularly to declining levels of productivity (Krugman 1996; Reich 1991). To remedy these problems, a concerted effort must be made to deal with the country's underlying economic weaknesses. In addition, Reich (1991) believes that existing educational and training approaches need to be reformed so that Americans will be better equipped to cope with the demands of the new 'information age'. He contends that the new economy demands a highly educated labour force comprised largely of 'symbolic analysts' rather than people with skills suited to the 'Fordist' industrial age. Reich recommends that educational programmes be expanded to create the human capital needed for Americans to compete successfully in the global economy.

However, these ideas are not universally accepted. Many Americans believe that market forces will resolve the economic difficulties the country has experienced over the last 20 years. Many also believe that these difficulties are the result of excessive state interference in the economy and a generous welfare system that impedes economic growth. They will hardly support additional government intervention. It is partly for this reason that American political leaders have been reluctant to adopt comprehensive, active labour market policies. Unlike European countries such as Sweden where the government intervenes to stimulate job creation and provide on-going skills training, many American policy makers believe that de-regulation and non-interference in the market offers the best prospect for future prosperity. The same attitudes characterise human capital development policies and programmes. Although the federal government has introduced various employment training programmes over the years, King (1995) reports that these programmes have been poorly funded and haphazardly implemented. A major problem is that they are perceived by employers as catering exclusively for social assistance recipients. Because of their low status, these trainees are stigmatised and unable to find work. Until these programmes focus on the population as a whole, they are likely to remain ineffective. The problem is exacerbated by the fact that American firms spend far less on worker training than their counterparts in Europe (Moore 1996).

Some writers argue that the problem of poverty in the United States (and other societies as well) should be dealt with through a comprehensive approach that emphasises economic and social development (Midgley 1995). State, market and community institutions need to be combined to promote a dynamic process of growth and social improvement. These ideas were reflected in a major study on poverty in the Lower Mississippi Valley (Lower Mississippi Delta Development Commission 1990). The study was designed to discover the causes of poverty and to make recommendations for its amelioration. The study paid particular attention to the need to harmonise economic development and social programmes. Although the Commission which directed the study was chaired by President Clinton, who was then governor of one of the region's states, he has not taken steps to implement its findings.

CONCLUSION: FUTURE TRENDS AND ISSUES

The different policy approaches used in America to combat poverty are the subject of on-going controversy. While there was previously greater consensus about the role of government in reducing poverty,

244 James Midgley and Michelle Livermore

attitudes have changed. Unlike the post-Second World War years, when government intervention was widely accepted, many political leaders now reject the idea that government should introduce poverty alleviation programmes. These programmes, they claim, are bound to fail. It is only when the market is permitted to operate free of government intervention that the economy will prosper and that employment and incomes will increase. This view is becoming increasingly popular in the United States.

Since the time of President Reagan, social programmes have been retrenched and the terms of the debate on poverty and social policy issues has changed dramatically (Midgley 1992; Glennerster 1991). The publication of books by intellectuals on the political right such as Gilder (1981), Murray (1984) and Mead (1986) have provided academic support for policy approaches that departed significantly from accepted ideas about the causes of poverty and the best ways of ameliorating it. The belief that poverty is due to personal inadequacy and that government policies have simply exacerbated the problem is now widely accepted. Despite the best efforts of progressive social scientists, these ideas now hold sway in political and in popular circles. These ideas have already resulted in the modification of conventional income-support policies.

As was noted earlier, the federal government has permitted many states to alter the AFDC programme by introducing a variety of eligibility requirements. These modifications have fostered a much more punitive approach to social assistance. The Republican Party's proposal that the whole AFDC programme be decentralised and that the states become responsible for social assistance is gradually being implemented. The enactment of the Personal Responsibility and Work Opportunity Reconciliation Act of 1996 is a major step in this direction. With the imposition of time limits and other requirements, the numbers of destitute people without any form of public support is likely to increase.

While social security is currently the subject of much media debate, few experts believe that major policy changes are likely in the near future. However, in view of the ideological nature of current criticisms of social security, major changes cannot be ruled out. Proposals for the introduction of privatised individual retirement accounts as an alternative to social security are already circulating in American policy circles.

Prevailing attitudes are also unlikely to produce major efforts by the federal government to promote community-based anti-poverty initiatives. While the enterprise zone programme introduced by the Clinton administration remains popular, the prospect of massive injections of federal resources for community-based economic development remains slim. The federal deficit also effectively impedes anti-poverty policy innovations of this kind. Indeed, efforts to reduce the deficit have also influenced current attempts to retrench the AFDC and other means-tested programmes.

Similarly, the present ideological climate is hardly conducive to significant federal intervention in the economy. The problem is exacerbated by the fact that economic policy is now largely determined by the Federal Reserve Bank, which has sought to curtail economic growth in order to prevent inflation. Its cautious stance is likely to result in relatively slow employment growth in the future.

The activist policies employed by previous administrations in an attempt to alleviate poverty are now only a historical phenomenon. Both the New Deal of the 1930s and War on Poverty of the 1960s are regularly vilified in right-wing circles. The idea that government intervention can successfully reduce poverty is scorned. These ideas are frequently restated in the media and public attitudes towards the poor have hardened. In this climate, the American poverty problem is likely to become even more acute and visible in the future.

REFERENCES

Abramovitz, M. (1995) 'Aid to Families with Dependent Children', in Edwards, R. *et al.* (eds) *Encyclopedia of Social Work* (19th edn), Washington, DC: National Association of Social Workers.

Becker, G. (1964) *Human Capital: A Theoretical and Empirical Analysis with Special Reference to Education*, New York: Columbia University Press.

Blakely, E. (1994) *Planning Local Economic Development: Theory and Practice*, Thousand Oaks, CA: Sage Publications.

Bluestone, B. and Harrison, B. (1982) *The Deindustrializing of America*, New York: Basic Books.

Bowles, S. and Gintis, H. (1976) *Schooling Capitalist America*, New York: Basic Books.

Danziger, S. and Gottschalk, P. (1995) *America Unequal*, Cambridge, MA: Harvard University Press.

Day, P. (1989) *A New History of Social Welfare*, Englewood Cliffs, NJ: Prentice Hall.

Etzioni, A. (1993) *The Spirit of Community: Rights, Responsibilities and the Communitarian Agenda*, New York: Crown Publishers.

Galaway, B. and Hudson, J. (eds) (1994) *Community Economic Development:*

Perspectives on Research and Policy, Toronto: Thompson Educational Publications.

Gilder, G. (1981) *Wealth and Poverty*, New York: Basic Books.

Glennerster, H. (1991) 'The Radical Right and the Future of the Welfare State', in Glennerster, H. and Midgley, J. (eds) *The Radical Right and the Welfare State: An International Assessment*, Savage, MD: Barnes and Noble.

Halpern, R. (1995) *Rebuilding the Inner City: A History of Neighborhood Initiatives to Address Poverty in the United States*, New York: Columbia University Press.

Harrington, M. (1962) *The Other America: Poverty in the United States*, New York: Macmillan.

King, D. (1995) *Actively Seeking Work: The Politics of Unemployment and Welfare Policy in the United States and Great Britain*, Chicago: University of Chicago Press.

Kingson, E.R. and Berkowitz, E.D. (1993) *Social Security and Medicare: A Policy Primer*, Westport, CT: Auburn House.

Krugman, P. (1996) *Pop Internationalism*. Cambridge, MA: MIT Press.

Leiby, J. (1978) *A History of Social Welfare and Social Work in the United States*, New York: Columbia University Press.

Lewis, O. (1966) 'The Culture of Poverty', *Scientific American* 214 (1): 19–25.

Lower Mississippi Delta Development Commission (1990) *The Delta Initiatives: Realizing the Dream, Fulfilling the Potential*, Memphis, TN: Lower Mississippi Delta Development Commission.

Massey, D.S. and Denton, N.A. (1993) *American Apartheid: Segregation and the Making of the Underclass*, Cambridge, MA: Harvard University Press.

Mead, L. (1986) *Beyond Entitlement: The Social Obligations of Citizenship*, New York: Basic Books.

—— (1996) 'Raising Work Levels Among the Poor', in Darby, M.R. (ed.) *Reducing Poverty in America: Views and Approaches*, Thousand Oaks, CA: Sage Publications.

Merton, R.K. (1957), *Social Theory and Social Structure*, New York: Free Press.

Midgley, J. (1992), 'Society, Social Policy and the Ideology of Reaganism', *Journal of Sociology and Social Welfare* 19 (1): 13–29.

—— (1995) *Social Development: The Developmental Perspective in Social Welfare*, Thousand Oaks, CA: Sage Publications.

Mondros, J.B. and Wilson, S. (1994) *Organizing for Power and Empowerment*, New York: Columbia University Press.

Moore, T.S. (1996) *The Disposable Workforce: Worker Displacement and Employment Instability in America*, New York: Aldine de Gruyter.

Murray, C. (1984) *Losing Ground: American Social Policy 1950–1980*, New York: Basic Books.

Murray, C. and Herrnstein, R.J. (1994) *The Bell Curve: Intelligence and Class Structure in American Society*, New York: Free Press.

Patterson, J.T. (1994) *America's Struggle Against Poverty 1900–1994*, Cambridge, MA: Harvard University Press.

Quadagno, J. (1994) *The Color of Welfare: How Racism Undermined the War on Poverty*, New York: Oxford University Press.

Reich, R. (1991) *The Work of Nations: Preparing Ourselves for 21st Century Capitalism*, New York: Alfred A. Knopf.

Rothman, D. and Rothman, S. (1972) *On Their Own: The Poor in Modern America*, Reading, MA: Addison-Wesley.

Schultz, T.W. (1960) 'Capital Formation by Education', *Journal of Political Economy* 68 (4): 571–83.

—— (1981) *Investing in People*, Berkeley, CA: University of California Press.

Segalman, R. and Asoke, B. (1981) *Poverty in America: The Welfare Dilemma*, Westport, CT: Greenwood Press.

Simon, B.L. (1994) *The Empowerment Tradition in American Social Work*, New York: Columbia University Press.

Skocpol, T. (1992) *Protecting Soldiers and Mothers: The Political Origins of Social Policy in the United States*, Cambridge, MA: Harvard University Press.

Townsend, P. (ed.) (1970) *The Concept of Poverty*, London: Heinemann Educational Books.

US, Bureau of the Census, (1975) *Historical Statistics of the United States*, Washington, DC: Bureau of the Census.

US, Bureau of the Census (1993) *Population of the United States: 1992*, (Current Population Reports, Series P60–185), Washington, DC: Bureau of the Census.

US, Bureau of the Census (1995) *Statistical Abstracts of the United States*, Washington, DC: Bureau of the Census.

US, Department of Health, Education and Welfare (1976) *The Measure of Poverty: A Report to Congress Mandated by the Education Amendments of 1974*, Washington, DC: Department of Health, Education and Welfare.

World Bank (1995) *World Tables*, Baltimore, MD: Johns Hopkins University Press.

Wilson, W.J. (1987) *The Truly Disadvantaged: The Inner City, the Underclass and Public Policy*, Chicago: University of Chicago Press.

Chapter 11

Zimbabwe

Edwin Kaseke

Zimbabwe (formerly Rhodesia) is located in southern Africa and became an independent sovereign state in April 1980. It had previously been a British colony since 1890, not withstanding the fact that the colony unilaterally declared independence from Britain in 1965. According to the most recent census (Zimbabwe 1992), Zimbabwe has a total population of 10.4 million of which 98.77 per cent are Africans, 0.80 per cent are European, with the remainder being Asians and persons of mixed races. The statistics also show that females constitute approximately 51 per cent of the total population. It is also noted from the same census report that 69 per cent of the population is classified as rural with 31 per cent classified as urban population. The annual population growth rate is 3.1 per cent and on average the population growth rate is higher in rural areas than in urban areas.

According to the United Nations Development Program (1994), Zimbabwe has an adult literacy rate of 69 per cent and a life expectancy of 56 years and those who have access to safe drinking water account for only 36 per cent of the population. The United Nations Development Program (1994) further reports that the per capita income was US$670 in 1991.

THE CHALLENGES OF A COLONIAL LEGACY

Before the advent of colonialism, the indigenous people depended on subsistence agriculture although there was also external trade in gold, ivory and copper (United Nations 1980: 8). Colonialism marked the turning point in the socio-economic profile of the country. The British South African Company, which wrested control of the territory from the indigenous people, was initially motivated by the hope of discovering huge gold deposits but later turned to agriculture, when they realised that their hopes had been misplaced. In order to protect the interests of the new settler community, the British South African Company moved swiftly to appropriate land from the indigenous population. In an effort to starve off competition from the indigenous farmers, the colonial settlers developed a policy of 'white supremacy' in agriculture which, according to Stoneman (1981), was realised through promoting the immigration of white farmers, offering low land prices and provision of credit facilities and agricultural extension services.

The policy of 'white supremacy' was given expression in the Land Apportionment Act of 1930 which divided land according to racial groups. The white settlers who at that time constituted approximately 3 per cent of the total population occupied 46.9 per cent of the land and most of it fell into the best agro-ecological regions. The Africans, on the other hand, were allocated 48.6 per cent of the land and this mainly fell into agro-ecological regions characterised by poor soils and low and erratic rainfall. This policy of white supremacy contributed significantly, to the marginalisation of the Africans and the peasant economy and was responsible for the dualism that came to characterise the economy of the country. The dualism reflected the existence of two different economic sub-systems namely the subsistence economy and a modern economy. The subsistence sector was a source of cheap labour for the modern economy. The wages were low and there were no social security schemes targeted at the indigenous workers. At the cessation of employment in the modern sector, African workers were expected to return to their rural homes.

At independence, the government sought to redress the imbalances of the past by integrating the peasant sector into the mainstream of the economy. Gibbon (1995: 7–8) observes that the shaping of socio-economic policies in Zimbabwe can be categorised into four phases. He argues that the first phase, from independence to 1982, was a phase of economic boom marked by redistributive policies whereas the second phase 1982 to 1985, was characterised by economic recession and a slowing down on redistributive policies. He goes on to argue that phase three 1985 to 1990, saw some level of economic growth but with a continued slowdown on redistributive policies, while phase four 1990 to 1994, was characterised by economic structural adjustment. The structural adjustment programme, which the government has been implementing since

1990, with the support of the International Monetary Fund and the World Bank, entails liberalising trade, adopting appropriate fiscal and monetary policies and deregulating the economy. The aim of this economic reform programme is to remove impediments to economic growth and thereby propel the country towards sustainable levels of economic growth.

POVERTY CONTEXTUALISED

The Government of Zimbabwe in its 1995 Poverty Assessment Study (Zimbabwe 1995a: iii) defines poverty in absolute terms as: 'the inability to afford a defined basket of consumption items (food and non-food) which are necessary to sustain life.'

There have been frequent studies to establish the poverty line in Zimbabwe in respect of African urban workers with a view to ensuring that wages are kept at a level high enough to meet the subsistence needs of workers. Cubitt and Riddell (1974: 5) defined the poverty line as: 'the income required to satisfy the minimum necessary consumption needs of a family of given size and composition within a defined environment in a condition of basic physical health and social decency'. They classified the items that were necessary to maintain physical health and social decency into nine categories; food, clothing, fuel and lighting, personal care and health, replacement of household goods, transport, accommodation, education and provision for post-employment consumption (Cubitt and Riddell 1974: 8). Despite the existence of a poverty line, the wages for the majority of African workers have always been below the poverty line.

The existence of relative poverty is often associated with highly unequal societies. Zimbabwe has serious disparities in the distribution of income and these disparities have a racial character. This was more pronounced before independence and as the United Nations (1980: 29) observes, 'the ratio of average real earnings of Europeans to those of Africans in the white economy has remained more or less constant at 11:1 throughout the entire post UDI [Unilateral Declaration of Independence] period [1965–80]'.

During the colonial period, Africans were treated as second class citizens and wages for African urban workers were based on rural subsistence rates. The assumption was that the needs of the Africans were simple and could not be compared to the sophistication associated with European needs. Income disparities are still evident in the 1990s although this is now a class issue.

POVERTY INCIDENCE

In order to understand the incidence of poverty in Zimbabwe, it is necessary to look at it from a historical perspective. The white settler regime introduced policies that were designed to promote and perpetuate their supremacy over the indigenous African population. Soon after independence, the average per capita incomes from peasant agriculture have been estimated by Riddell (1981: 53) to range from Z$25 to Z$30 per annum (Riddell 1981: 53). Riddell further points out that these incomes were too low to sustain rural families and their survival was only enhanced by cash or in-kind transfers from employed relatives. The rural areas are still characterised by low incomes largely because the problem of land shortage still remains and because agricultural operations are still seasonal. Furthermore, Zimbabwe has been experiencing frequent droughts and given the vulnerability of peasant farmers, the viability of the peasant sector has been seriously affected.

By 1985, the economy of Zimbabwe had begun to send distress signals. These distress signals were reflected in a growing budget deficit of about 10 per cent of Gross Domestic Product (GDP) and a growing government debt which by 1989 had reached a peak of 71 per cent of GDP (Sachikonye 1995: 42–3). In response to the economic crisis, the government decided to implement its economic structural adjustment programme.

The structural adjustment programme has had a negative impact on the welfare of the people due to its transitional costs. These include sharp increases in the prices of basic commodities and services which make it difficult for the poor to access goods and services that are crucial for the satisfaction of their basic needs. The price increases at the initial stages are largely due to the removal of subsidies on basic commodities in an effort to reduce the budget deficit. The transitional costs also include cost-recovery measures in the form of user-fees in the areas of health and education. The introduction of user-fees has resulted in reduced utilisation of health facilities and an increase in the number of school drop-outs.

According to the 1995 Poverty Assessment Study (Zimbabwe 1995a), 62 per cent of the country's population belong to households whose incomes are inadequate to meet basic needs. The study also revealed that 42 per cent of the households are below the 'food poverty line' and the study concluded that the incidence of poverty is greater in rural areas where 72 per cent of households have incomes below the 'total consumption poverty line' compared to 46 per cent in urban areas. The 'total consumption poverty line' indicates the income needed to purchase food and non-food needs of a family of a given size whereas the food poverty line focuses on the income needed to purchase food only.

POVERTY PROFILE

The groups that are most affected by poverty include the unemployed, low income earners, the informal sector workers, peasant farmers and women – particularly single-parents as the following discussion will show.

The unemployed and informal sector workers

The problem of unemployment in Zimbabwe has its roots in the colonial policy of deliberately marginalising African agriculture. Riddell (1981: 158) observes that: 'Decades of neglect of the peasant sector resulting in increased numbers of people offering themselves for work in the modern sectors of the economy at very low levels of remuneration has not achieved anything like full employment.'

The problem of unemployment continues to worsen and it is estimated to stand at 40 per cent in the mid-1990s. The problem is worsening because of the economy's inability to generate more jobs in the face of a growing population. The economy is able to generate about 17,000 jobs per year yet there are about 300,000 persons entering the job market every year. The problem of unemployment has also worsened because of structural adjustment-induced retrenchment of workers. By the mid-1990s, a total of 60,000 workers from both the private and public sectors had been retrenched.

In the absence of a comprehensive social security system, the unemployed find themselves without any meaningful safety net. They are then forced to engage in a variety of survival strategies including participation in the informal sector. Common activities in the informal sector include the sale of fruits, vegetables, embroidery and second-hand clothing. Whilst the informal sector provides opportunities for earning income, the incomes are, however, generally low and thus making it difficult for workers to meet their basic needs. Furthermore, informal sector workers still experience constraints such as harassment by the police and lack of access to credit facilities.

Low income earners

Low income earners in both the private and public sectors comprise mostly of unskilled and semi-skilled workers. The incomes of these workers are often below the poverty line and because, with high levels of unemployment, there is no pressure on employers to pay adequate wages. At independence, the government took upon itself to determine minimum wages for the different sectors and thereby forcing employers to pay reasonable wages. In many instances, however, minimum wages were set below the poverty line and the government's argument was that it had to balance poverty ameliora-tion with the need to safeguard existing jobs by taking cognisance of the employers' capacity to pay higher wages.

This low-wages policy serves to condemn many workers to a life of poverty. It is almost impossible for them to accumulate any savings or to take up private insurance to protect their meagre stan-dard of living in the event of old age, disability and so forth. This problem is most acute among domestic workers and farm workers. For instance, it is most evident that malnutrition is higher among children of farm workers.

Peasant farmers

The peasant sector has historically been disadvantaged owing to the colonial policies which sought to promote white agriculture at the expense of the indigenous majority. The land used by the majority of the peasants is not fertile and continues to deteriorate because of overuse. The overcrowding which has occurred because of popula-tion growth has forced families to subdivide their land in order to ensure that every male child has access to land. Subdividing the land has, however, made the landholdings too small and therefore uneconomic. The productivity of peasant farmers is still being hampered by limited access to credit facilities occasioned by a lending system which is not well suited to the circumstances of the peasants. Furthermore, there is lack of draught power since cattle herds were greatly depleted during the liberation war and were further depleted after independence because of the successive droughts.

Women

African women have traditionally been disadvantaged owing to cultural practices that designated the roles of women as those of 'child bearing, child rearing, washing clothes, fetching water, cooking and working in the fields' (Riddell 1981:43). Traditionally, women were considered minors and were not expected to make major decisions. At independence, the government sought to improve the status of women by enacting the Legal Age of Majority Act in 1982, which gave majority status to both males and females on attaining the age of 18 years. This has also resulted in equal pay for equal work regardless of sex.

Although legislation exists to promote the status of women, the marginalisation of women still persists. In the rural areas, for instance, women have no entitlement to land in their own right even though they are the ones who work the land. Most of the women do not make major decisions on their own. They either wait for their husbands to return from the urban areas or refer matters to the male relatives of their husbands. In many instances, incomes accrued from their farming operations have to be surrendered to their husbands resulting in women not benefiting from the fruits of their labour.

Single mothers are particularly vulnerable to poverty and according to the Ministry of National Affairs, Employment Creation and Cooperatives (Zimbabwe 1995b: 36), poverty in female-headed households: 'may be due to a more limited access to land for widows and divorcees compared to married women, and a more limited access to agricultural resources and labour'. In urban areas, women dominate the informal sector and while married women use the informal sector to supplement their husbands' incomes, single-mothers use it as their only source of income.

SOCIAL WELFARE RESPONSES TO POVERTY

The social welfare system is based on the residual model and is a product of the country's racial history where it predominantly served the interests of the white community (Hampson and Kaseke 1987). The social welfare system targets the most needy members of society and assistance is supposed to be withdrawn as soon as beneficiaries are able to draw support from the market economy or their families. The major social welfare responses to poverty in Zimbabwe include public assistance, drought relief and the Social Development Fund.

Public assistance programme

The public assistance programme established in 1964 was designed to address the problem of poverty and its primary objective is 'to relieve distress and to rehabilitate those permanently or temporarily disadvantaged' (Riddell 1981: 172). During the colonial period, public assistance for Africans was restricted to those who were permanent urban residents (Gargett 1977: 67). Gargett (1977: 67) further observes that non-urbanised Africans living in urban areas were repatriated to their rural homes on the assumption that the peasant economy had the capacity to look after its own destitute.

Public assistance in the mid-1990s is provided in terms of the Welfare Assistance Act of 1988 and is provided to indigent persons who fall in the following categories of persons:

- persons over the age of 60 years;
- persons with physical or mental disabilities;
- persons who suffer from chronic illness; and
- dependents of indigent persons.

Public assistance is only provided to persons who can show that they do not have the income necessary to sustain themselves and their families. This means-tested assistance is granted only in circumstances where individuals are unable to secure assistance from their families and where they have no other sources of income. Furthermore, the payment of public assistance is restricted to the citizens of Zimbabwe only. Foreign nationals are only assisted pending repatriation to their countries.

Although rehabilitation of the poor is an important objective of the public assistance programme, this is not being achieved because the benefits provided are too low to propel beneficiaries towards self-reliance let alone to enable them to meet their basic needs. Furthermore, the resources allocated for public assistance are too low to support the growing population of needy or destitute people. Consequently, there is a high degree of selectivity in the provision of public assistance resulting in very few people benefiting from the programme. Approximately one person in every twenty needy persons is probably being assisted by public assistance (Kaseke 1993: 86).

It should also be pointed out that public assistance's urban bias remains. There are a number of factors that explain this bias. First, the social welfare offices in urban areas are usually located within easy reach of the people. Consequently, it is easier for urban residents to access assistance. Second, people in urban areas have more access to information and they are therefore more aware of the services provided than their rural counterparts. Lastly, absolute poverty is still viewed as an urban phenomenon particularly given the fact that urban people have to pay for their housing, water, electricity and food and as a result applications from urban residents are more readily approved.

Social insurance

In the early 1980s, the government declared its intention to introduce a comprehensive social insurance system in order to provide income protection against major contingencies. At the top of government priority was the need to introduce a social insurance scheme that would provide income protection against the contingency of old age. This was based on the understanding that many workers were retiring without any income protection to enable them to meet their post-retirement needs. Consequently, most retired workers found themselves in poverty. Although some retired workers were receiving occupational pensions, the pensions were usually inadequate, rendering the retired workers unable to meet their basic needs.

The government finally introduced the Pensions and Other Benefits Scheme which became operational in October 1994. The scheme is contributory, with employees contributing 3 per cent of their insurable earnings up to a ceiling of Z$4,000 per month with the employers matching the contributions of their employees. The scheme provides for retirement benefit, death benefit, survivors benefit and invalidity benefit. The benefits paid depend on the employee's level of contributions except for the death benefit which is set at a flat rate.

The effectiveness of this scheme as an anti-poverty programme is undermined by the fact that it only covers a minority of the population. At present the scheme does not cover civil servants, workers in some semi-public enterprises, domestic workers, informal sector workers and peasants. Furthermore, there is concern that the rate of contribution and the ceiling of insurable earnings are too low to guarantee the viability of the scheme and too low to guarantee adequacy of benefits.

Rural drought relief

Another social welfare response to poverty is the provision of rural drought relief to the victims of drought. The drought relief is specifically geared towards meeting the food requirements of the victims of drought. It is provided only to those who are wholly dependent on agriculture for their sustenance and thus excludes families whose breadwinners are employed in the formal sector. The lists of eligible persons are compiled by the local community leadership.

In order to avoid the development of a dependence syndrome, the government introduced the Food-for-Work Programme in 1989. This involved victims of drought working on community projects in return for food. The Public Works Programme introduced before independence, was also utilised and enabled victims of drought to work on community projects in return for cash which they would use to purchase food. Only vulnerable groups, such as the elderly and the chronically ill, were not expected to work for their food. The Food-for-Work and Public Works Programmes have not been able to cater for all eligible persons in the communities because of the small-scale nature of these projects. The government introduced the Grain Loan Scheme in 1994 whereby the rural people are loaned grain on condition that they will repay it at the next harvest. However, vulnerable groups continue to receive free drought relief.

It is too early to evaluate the Grain Loan Scheme as it has just started. However, it remains to be seen whether the government has the administrative capacity to enable it to follow-up repayments. The major weakness of both the Drought Relief Programme and Grain Loan Scheme is that their focus is on meeting the food requirements but ignore the other areas of consumption.

Social Development Fund

After the introduction of the Economic Structural Adjustment Programme in October 1990, the government set up the Social Development Fund with a welfare component designed to cushion the poor and vulnerable groups against the negative effects of structural adjustment. The target groups are the low income earners, retrenched workers and the unemployed. The welfare component of the Social Development Fund provides assistance with the payment of school fees and medical/hospital fees for persons with monthly household incomes of Z$400 or less and also initially offered food subsidies to persons with monthly household incomes not exceeding Z$200. Food subsidies were later withdrawn allegedly because the administrative costs were unduly burdensome. Furthermore, the amounts awarded were small and as a result the take-up rate was low. The impact of the Social Development Fund in cushioning the poor has been minimal because of the weaknesses in the design and implementation of the Fund (Kaseke 1994). First, the system of using household incomes instead of per capita incomes within households has meant that the safety nets have been unable to capture the most needy persons. Second, applicants have to travel long distances in order to lodge applications with their nearest social welfare office and this disadvantages the rural poor as the offices in the rural areas are not within easy reach of the majority of the people. Thus, the services are not easily accessible to the rural poor.

ANTI-POVERTY PROGRAMME

At independence, the government acknowledged that the problem of poverty in rural areas was due to landlessness, overcrowding and lack of access to credit facilities. The government therefore took the following measures in order to arrest the problem of poverty.

Land reform

It was agreed at the Lancaster House Agreement in 1979 that the government would resettle those with inadequate land and the landless people on land purchased by the government on a 'willing seller, willing buyer' basis. The pace of resettlement however, has been very slow as evidenced by the fact that by early 1989 only 45,000 families had been resettled (Kaseke 1993: 77). This slow pace was largely attributed to the unwillingness of commercial farmers to sell their land and to the inability of government to mobilise the necessary resources to purchase the farms.

Critics of the resettlement programme have pointed out that those who have been resettled have failed to utilise the land productively and fear that this will impact negatively on the country's food security. There is no doubt, however, that the government felt constrained by the principle of 'willing seller, willing buyer'. It is therefore not surprising that in 1992, the government enacted the Land Acquisition Act which empowers the President to designate land which can be used for resettlement purposes. The farmers whose land is designated receive compensation from the government. By the mid-1990s, 3.37 million hectares of land have been purchased and 62,000 families resettled. Although, according to the Land Acquisition Act, the President can designate any land, the government has however made a commitment not to designate land which is being fully utilised in order to avoid undermining the country's food security. In the same vein, the government also pledged to resettle only those farmers who are able to use the land productively.

Despite the enactment of the Land Acquisition Act, the problems of landlessness and overcrowding in the rural areas still persist. The government seems to be moving cautiously amid accusations from white commercial farmers that land designation is a violation of human rights and that it is using designation as a political weapon. The fact, remains however, that unless government expedites the land redistribution process, the marginalisation of the rural people will continue.

Institutional support for peasant farmers

Prior to independence, the Agricultural Finance Corporation never provided credit facilities to the peasant farmers. The new majority government recognised the need to extend credit facilities to the peasant farmers and the value of loans disbursed to peasant farmers rose from Z\$4.2 million in 1980 to Z\$60 million in 1986 (Kaseke 1993: 73).

Access to credit facilities enabled peasant farmers, for the first time, to buy essential agricultural inputs such as fertilisers, pesticides and improved seed varieties. Although access to credit facilities improved the productive capacity of the peasant farmers, there are a number of problems associated with the lending system. The major one encountered by the farmers is that almost all the income derived form the sale of their produce goes towards servicing the loans obtained from the Agricultural Finance Corporation. This has tended to discourage farmers from borrowing from the Agricultural Finance Corporation which could result in reduced productivity owing to no or limited application of fertilisers. Some farmers try to avoid loan repayments by selling their produce to middlemen instead of selling directly to the Grain Marketing Board, which has an arrangement with the Agricultural Finance Corporation for automatic loan deductions. The situation has now been exacerbated by the deregulation in the marketing of grain which no longer obliges farmers to sell their grain to the Grain Marketing Board. The default rate in the repayment of loans has increased to the point of threatening the viability of the Agricultural Finance Corporation itself.

The other institutional support measure was the decision by government to establish marketing depots within easy reach of the farmers. Prior to this, many peasants were incurring considerable transport costs in moving their produce to the marketing boards. Although decentralisation has reduced the distances that peasant farmers have to travel in order to sell their produce, the roads are often poorly maintained, a situation which forces transporters to charge exorbitant rates.

In view of the problems that have been highlighted, there is need for the government to take a holistic approach to the problem of poverty in the rural areas. The productive capacities of the peasant farmers can not be fully utilised unless concerted efforts are made to harness water for irrigation purposes given the fact that Zimbabwe has rainy and dry seasons. The majority of peasant farmers utilise their land for at most six months in a year and both the land and the farmers are idle for the other six months. The development of irrigation facilities would greatly improve the incomes of the peasants and ultimately improve the quality of life.

Employment creation

With the unemployment rate around 40 per cent, it is a social problem which has also been exacerbated by the economic structural adjustment programme being implemented by the government. Retrenchment of workers in both the private and public sector continues to be a major characteristic of that programme.

The government launched the Employment and Training Program in 1992 as a component of the Social Development Fund set up to cushion the people particularly the 'new poor' against the adverse effects of structural adjustment. The objective of employment programme is to generate employment both short-term and long-term. The generation of short-term employment focuses on the labour-intensive public works projects which are designed to improve the physical infrastructure of communities. Long-term employment generation on the other hand, focuses on promoting small-scale enterprises with potential for growth. This programme is primarily intended to give retrenched workers a new lease of life. Retrenched workers are required to submit project ideas to designated consultants after receiving training. The consultants would then prepare project proposals on behalf of the retrenched workers. These are submitted to the Coordinating Unit of the Social Development Fund for appraisal.

Although about 60,000 workers have been retrenched, only a few have been able to start small-to-medium scale enterprises. By the end of June 1996, a total of 1,941 projects had been approved at a cost of Z$158 million. These projects generated a total of 7,435 jobs. These statistics show that only a few retrenched workers have utilised this facility. Some retrenchees were not aware of this facility and others just failed to develop project proposals. Some of the enterprises have not been successful owing to a variety of factors which include poor business management and stiff competition from established businesses. The disbursement of funds for employment creation has been very slow and this has tended to upset the business plans of retrenched workers. Furthermore, because of price escalations, input costs continue to rise making the disbursements inadequate to guarantee viability of the small-to-medium scale enterprises.

An important point to note is that the Employment and Training Programme was designed on the assumption that retrenched workers will have received their retrenchment packages (severance pay) in accordance with the conditions for retrenchment. Retrenched workers are expected to contribute at least 10 per cent of the total loan value, yet there are numerous reports of retrenchment workers who never received their retrenchment packages. As a result, retrenched workers who did not receive their retrenchment packages find it difficult to raise the 10 per cent contribution required. Consequently, such retrenched workers never benefit from the Employment and Training Programme.

Chemwanyisa (1993) in a study of the Employment and Training Programme, observes that a significant number of retrenched workers were either illiterate or semi-literate and were therefore unable to benefit fully from the training offered. Consequently, such people had problems in developing project ideas. Chemwanyisa (1993) further observes that retrenchments have often resulted in

trauma as these are usually effected suddenly with little or no preparation on the part of the workers. This problem is compounded by
the attitudes of some retrenchees who are easily intimidated by the
procedures involved in setting up small businesses. Such people
would rather wait for another opportunity to be employed than
start their own businesses.

The Employment and Training Programme could have made a
greater national impact if it had not confined itself to assisting
retrenched workers only. This limitation is reflective of the preoccupation of economies under structural adjustment with the 'new
poor'. There is need to bring in the 'old poor' as well since the
Structural Adjustment Programme worsens their poverty.

FUTURE PROSPECTS AND STRATEGIES

The Government of Zimbabwe developed the Poverty Alleviation
Action Plan towards the end of 1993 to provide a framework for the
reduction of poverty. According to the Ministry of Public Service,
Labour and Social Welfare (Zimbabwe 1994: 3) the following
initiatives would be undertaken:

- mobilising civil society through awareness campaigns and
  capacity building;
- upgrading infrastructure and services in rural communities;
- creation of small-scale enterprises; and
- developing appropriate social safety nets to cushion the poor.

In principle, the Poverty Alleviation Action Plan offers quite a
comprehensive approach to the problem of poverty and unemployment. The major issue of concern however, is that it relies heavily
on international aid for its implementation. Thus, if the donors
were to withdraw their support, the Plan would prove difficult to
implement. There is no indication in the Plan of how the government will build its own capacity to implement the Plan with little
or no support from international aid agencies. Furthermore, the
strategies given in the Plan are not new at all and it is not clear how
these strategies would produce the desired results this time.

In view of the magnitude of poverty in Zimbabwe, there is also
need for the government to mobilise resources in order to make it
possible for the public assistance programme to respond effectively
to the needs of the poor. Furthermore, it is necessary to ensure that

public assistance is not seen as an end in itself but rather as a means through which individuals can meet their basic needs whilst, at the same time, providing a medium through which self-reliance can be achieved. There is therefore a need to link public assistance to employment creation, so as to provide the poor with the means to earn income in a sustainable manner.

CONCLUSION

The reduction of poverty will remain an elusive goal unless the government addresses, in a holistic manner, the marginalisation of the rural people. To begin with, the land redistribution process needs to be expedited. The government needs to mobilise resources for the purchase of land and it is estimated that the government needs about Z1 billion for this purpose. It is also necessary to improve the lending system of the Agricultural Finance Corporation so as to make it more responsive to the needs of peasant farmers. Furthermore, it is important to improve the marketing of produce by the peasant farmers with a view to ensuring that they do not fall prey to middlemen who are preventing them from realising better returns on their production. An improvement in the quality of life in rural areas is likely to stem the tide of rural-urban migration.

Although the Structural Adjustment Programme is intended to revitalise the economy, the transitional costs that impact negatively on the poor do not appear transitional at all. In the absence of an alternative economic reform programme, it is important to improve the targeting of social safety nets in order to capture the poor. Furthermore, employment creation through developing small and medium scale enterprises should not be confined to the 'new poor' but should be extended to the 'old poor' as well.

REFERENCES

Chemwanyisa, N.S. (1993) 'An Assessment of the Employment and Training Program of Retrenched Workers' (an unpublished Bachelor of Social Work Dissertation), Harare: School of Social Work, University of Zimbabwe.

Cubitt, V. and Riddell, R. (1974) *The Urban Poverty Datum Line In Rhodesia*, Salisbury: Faculty of Social Studies, University of Rhodesia.

Gargett, E. (1977) *The Administration of Transition: African Urban Settlement in Rhodesia*, Gael: Mambo Press.

Gibbon, P. (1995) 'Introduction: Structural Adjustment and the Working

Poor in Zimbabwe', in Gibbon, P. (ed.) *Structural Adjustment and the Working Poor in Zimbabwe*, Uppsala: Nordiska Afrikainstitutet.

Hampson, J. and Kaseke, E. (1987) 'Zimbabwe', in Dixon, J. (ed.) *Social Welfare in Africa*, London: Croom Helm.

Kaseke, E. (1993) *Rural Social Security Needs: The Case of Zimbabwe*, Harare: School of Social Work.

—— (1994) *A Situation Analysis of the Social Development Fund* (Occasional Paper Series No. 2), Harare: School of Social Work.

Riddell, R. (1981) *Report of the Commission of Inquiry into Incomes, Prices and Conditions of Service*, Harare: Government Printer.

Sachikonye, L.M. (1995) 'Industrial Relations and Labour Relations Under ESAP in Zimbabwe', in Gibbon, P. (ed.) *Structural Adjustment and the Working Poor in Zimbabwe*, Uppsala: Nordiska Afrikainstitutet.

Stoneman, C. (1981),'Agriculture', in Stoneman, C. (ed.) *Zimbabwe's Inheritance*, London: The Macmillan Press.

United Nations (1980) *Zimbabwe: Towards a New Order*, New York: United Nations.

United Nations Development Program (1994) *Human Development Report*, New York: Oxford University Press.

Zimbabwe (1992) *Census; Zimbabwe National Report*, Harare: Central Statistical Office.

—— (1994) *Implementation of the Poverty Alleviation Action Plan*, Harare: Ministry of Public Service, Labour and Social Welfare.

—— (1995a) *Poverty Assessment Study Survey: Preliminary Report*, Harare: Ministry of Public Service, Labour and Social Welfare.

—— (1995b) *The Zimbabwe National Report For The Fourth World Conference on Women*, Harare: Ministry of National Affairs, Employment Creation and Co-operatives.

Chapter 12

Poverty in review

David Macarov and John Dixon

SUMMARY

Although the ten countries reviewed on in this volume are neither a random nor a representative sample, they are nevertheless illustrative in their diversity, as their size and population data in Table 12.1 indicates.

Economically, most are highly industrialised and/or urbanised countries, although agrarian populations dominate in the Philippines and Zimbabwe. Some have emerged from colonial

Table 12.1 Diversity of size of countries reviewed

Country	Area (km²)	Population*
Australia	7,687,000	18,000,000
Canada	10,000,000	29,000,000
Hong Kong	1,000	6,000,000
Ireland	69,000	3,500,000
Malta	300	350,000
Netherlands	41,000	15,500,000
Philippines	300,000	67,000,000
United Kingdom	240,000	59,000,000
United States	9,160,000	265,000,000
Zimbabwe	380,000	10,400,000

Note:
* Figures rounded.

status rather recently – Hong Kong, Malta, Philippines and Zimbabwe – while the others either had long cast aside their colonial yokes or have never been under foreign domination. The industrialised countries reviewed have long-standing and well-developed social welfare programmes, while others have only plans, or rudimentary social welfare institutions. Finally, as indicated in Table 12.2, some use relative definitions of poverty, some use absolute definitions, and some supplement their definitions with subjective investigations.

Regardless of the defining method used, the poverty rate in the highly industrialised and/or urbanised countries reviewed ranges from 7.1 per cent to 25 per cent of the population, while in the basically agricultural countries, it ranges from 40 per cent to 70 per cent.

The poverty profiles of the countries reviewed are summarised in Table 12.3. In eight of the ten countries, the elderly are a group in poverty; or, conversely, amongst those in poverty are the elderly.

Table 12.2 The percentage of relative, absolute and subjective poverty in the ten countries reviewed

	Relative poverty (%)	Absolute poverty (%)	Subjective poverty (%)
Australia	16.4	–	–
Canada	16.6	–	–
Hong Kong	–	15.5	–
Ireland	7–35*	–	–
Malta	10–15	–	11.8
Netherlands	7.1	–	11.1
Philippines	–	40–70	–
United Kingdom	25.0	–	–
United States	–	15.1	–
Zimbabwe	–	62.0	–

Note:
* Using various cut-off points.

The next most often mentioned group are single parents, primarily single-mothers. It is not always clear whether these are unmarried mothers, divorcees, or widows, but the presumption is that they cannot work because they are taking care of children, and therefore are in poverty. This is evidently part of the reasons why the next most often mentioned group in poverty are children. The low-paid worker and the unemployed share equally in the next rank of reasons given for poverty, followed by farmers and the disabled. Immigrants, disabled people and indigenous groups are also mentioned as among the groups in poverty.

Anti-poverty programmes specifically designed and implemented to alleviate or eradicate poverty exist only in four of the ten countries reviewed, although all have adopted strategies that impact on poverty, directly or indirectly, intentionally or unintentionally, as can be seen in Table 12.4.

The most-often cited strategy effecting poverty is social security (including social (general) assistance). The next most-often mentioned strategy is job creation, or efforts to arrive at full employment. Subsidies for housing, or housing improvements, are utilised in four countries, while plans for promoting economic development are seen as aiding the poor in three countries.

In summary, despite the differences between the countries

Table 12.3 The frequency of groups in poverty in the ten countries reviewed

Population group	Inclusion in national poverty profiles (% of countries reviewed)
The elderly	80
Single parents	70
Children	60
Working poor	60
Unemployed	60
Farmers	40
Disabled	30
Immigrants	20
Indigenous people	20

Table 12.4: The social policy strategies adopted in the ten countries
reviewed

Strategies	Adoption by country (% of countries reviewed)
Social security	90
Full employment/job creation	50
Housing subsidies/improvements	40
Macroeconomic/economic development	30
Training and retraining programmes	30
Empowerment of the poor/local community development	30
Agrarian land reform	20
Social development	20
Provisions for child care	10
Seed money for entrepreneurs	10
Credit banks	10
Population management	10
Minimum wages	10
Changes in tax policy	10
Reducing bureaucracy	10
Charity	10

reviewed in this volume, and the different methods they use to
define poverty, the groups most frequently living in poverty are the
elderly, single-parents, children, the working poor, and the unemployed, and that the most popular measures adopted that directly or
indirectly impact on poverty are social security and job creation,
although poverty alleviation or elimination may not always their
primary intent.

CONCLUSION

The poor are not merely statistics

Poverty can be defined in many ways, ranging from lack of the barest necessities for subsistence to an uncomfortable feeling of social exclusion or powerlessness. It can also be measured in a number of ways: by pre- and post-transfer income; by assets; by expenditures; by activities or their lack; by self-reports and by hypothetical questions. The units used can be the individual, the family unit, or differentially-defined family units. The poverty line can be drawn using absolute, relative, subjective or normative criteria. Despite all these definitional differences, poverty in the ten countries reviewed here affects from 7 to 25 people in every hundred in the highly industrial and/or urban countries, and twice or more that rate in the predominantly agricultural countries. Insofar as changes in poverty figures over time are reported in this volume, they remain within this range. Yet poverty data cannot be accepted uncritically.

Substantial reservoirs of hidden poor have been detected in many national studies. Room (1993: 110) describes them in the European setting as:

> Those who do not apply for social assistance . . . ; people who are missed by official surveys, such as single homeless and clandestine immigrants; women and children who suffer as a result of intra-household maldistribution of resources; and people who are confined in institutions.

Callan and Nolan (Chapter 5) report that the extent of poverty is under-reported in official figures in Ireland.

There is also the fact that given a choice of definitions or methods of measurement, governments almost invariably choose those that report the lowest number of poor people. For example, Dirven, Fouarge and Muffels (Chapter 7) point out that politicians and their constituents tend to differ as to what constitutes minimum subsistence. Similarly, the American poverty line mentioned by MacPherson and Silburn (Chapter 1) was originally based upon a food budget intended to cover an emergency period of only four days, but is now used without that restriction (Macarov 1970).

In addition to those people defined as poor, there is the stratum referred to as the 'near poor' – that is, those who are on the edge of poverty, or just above the poverty line, whose lives are marked by insecurity and fear of decreased income. In the United States, there are almost twice as many near poor as there are poverty-stricken (Roper 1991: 39), and as Tabone (Chapter 6) mentions, there may be as many as 50 per cent of Maltese households that are verging on relative poverty.

For those officially defined as poor. poverty is not simply a statistical artefact. It is, in Gans's (1967: 110) words, 'face-grinding, belly-gripping' poverty. Or, as a United Nations (UN 1995: 7) puts it: 'a condition of life so limited by malnutrition, illiteracy, disease, squalid surroundings, high infant mortality, and low life expectancy as to be below any reasonable definition of human decency.'

It is under these circumstances that more than one-fifth of the world's population now lives – that is, on less than one US$1 a day (UN 1995: 7).

The treatment of the poor in history

Poverty has deep historical roots. As early as 2370 BC a Sumerian ruler is reported to have tried to curb the oppression of the poor by officials and priests (*Encyclopaedia Britannica* 1965, 11: 41), and almost every religion dating from ancient times enjoins its followers to engage in charity, in some cases with the amounts and methods clearly outlined (Levenberg 1994). In Christianity, one is told that there is 'faith, hope and charity – and the greatest of these is charity'. When Jews gather on Yom Kippur to atone for their collective sins, they repeat, 'Prayer, repentance and charity will avert an evil decree'. In Islam, there is an obligatory tax (*zakat*) for the poor and needy, and during Ramadan each Moslem is required to feed at least one poor person (Dixon 1987).

Poverty has sometimes been caused by general lack of resources affecting almost the entire population, as when the potato crop failed in Ireland in the 1840s or during the Great Depression in 1930s. It has sometimes been due to individual tribulations, such as crippling of the chief earner, or the advent of single-parenthood. And sometimes it has been caused by inequity in resource distribution, as when the monarch or the church appropriated property and/or income, or when the economic system favours the upper echelons of the socio-economic spectrum at the expense of the lowest levels.

Whether due to the exhortations of ancient prophets, the activities of modern social reformers or occasional rulers or lawmakers, there have often been attempts to alleviate poverty, if not to eliminate it. The Bible forbade the gleaning of fields and the harvesting of corners in order to provide for the poor. Religious orders, monasteries and churches undertook to care for the poor during the Middle Ages. In Speenhamland, England, in 1795, a wage-supplement scheme to combat poverty was adopted by the local government – a programme, incidentally, which had to be abandoned due to the avarice of employers, not of the poor (Macarov 1970: 10–12). In the 1960s the United States government mounted a well-publicised War on Poverty, and since then the United Nations has declared a year devoted to concentration on poverty. However, no such programmes or measures have ever commanded enough resources, facilities and public support to have a widespread impact. In the United States, for example, Silver and Silver (1991: 321) point out: 'Since 1981 there has been no War on Poverty – it is as if victory had been declared, when in fact there was no such conquest.'

Indeed, as President Reagan is said to have remarked, 'We declared war on poverty, and poverty won.'

The persistence of poverty despite often considerable policy efforts

While only four of the countries reviewed in the volume have programmes directed intentionally at relieving poverty, and while Shewell's sobering view (Chapter 3) that in Canada 'the will to alleviate/minimise poverty through state intervention has been largely abandoned' may well have considerably broader applicability, all ten countries reviewed have adopted strategies to address some element of their perceived poverty 'problem', even if only as a unintended side-effect. The operative question is why, in the face of such varied and often long-continued policy effort, is poverty so persistent?

Reasons advanced for the continued existence of poverty are varied Macarov (1970: 10–12). One underlying reason sometimes posited is that the Biblical comment, 'the poor ye will always have with you' is interpreted by many to mean that attempts to eliminate poverty are contrary to God's will; or that the existence of poverty is pre-ordained and therefore must be accepted without question or counter-activity. Taken further, the poor are thus necessary so that the non-poor can gain merit in heaven by helping them, and carried even further, by some, there is perceived merit in being poor.

Another possibility that has been advanced is that the existence of poor people offers a sense of superiority to the non-poor – a sense that they are reluctant to give up. There is also the view that poverty is the whiplash which drives people to work – that is, a necessary spur to effort. Tabone (Chapter 6) puts this succinctly: if those on social assistance are brought to the same standard of living as those gainfully employed, 'This would lead to lack of initiative on the part of the citizen'.

Then there is the social Darwinist reasoning that if people are poor it must be their own fault, and therefore they should suffer the consequences (Macarov 1995: 209–10). Flowing from this is the generalisation that poor people are simply lazy and – a further step – would rather be poor than to do anything about it, including taking advantage of opportunities to improve their lot – an imputation which has been termed, 'blaming the victim' (Ryan 1974), which was punctured by Goodwin (1972) long ago.

In contrast to imputing poverty to personal inadequacy, there have been and are those who see poverty as a product of the dynamics of the socio-economic system. And, of course, there are combinations of these views, not always consistent with one another.

Finally, it would not do to ignore the implications of sexism, racism and xenophobia in creating and maintaining poverty. The feminisation of poverty has been noted by a number of researchers (for example, Room 1993; Abramovitz 1993), the unequal proportion of non-whites in poverty in predominately white countries is well documented, and the plight of new immigrants constitutes one of the normative aspects of poverty in most countries. Arising from these views and inconsistencies are the various programmes attempted and proposed in this volume.

The inadequacy of social security as an anti-poverty strategy

Social security is overwhelmingly intended to prevent the middle classes from falling into poverty, not to take people out of poverty (Dixon 1996b). It embraces retirement, disability and survivors' pensions, unemployment compensation, workplace injury and death benefits, sickness and maternity benefits, and children's and family allowances. In order to be eligible for such programmes, persons must be covered by them, which means largely those who have held full-time, permanent jobs in the formal sector. Then comes the almost universal principle of the 'wage stop,' which holds that no one should be able to acquire from social security more income than he or she would acquire by working, even if they are out of the workforce for reasons of age or disability or are unable to find work (Macarov 1980). Pensions and benefits are usually modest percentages of average wages, average incomes, or last salaries, even contribution-related lump sums. This means that those whose careers are marked by low-paying jobs, part-time work, work in the informal sector, and many or long periods of unemployment or periods out of the workforce usually receive the lowest level of income support (Macarov 1980; Dixon 1994, 1996a; Midgley 1993). So if this is their only source of income those at the lower end of the payment spectrum may well remain in poverty line. Consequently, those who were poor while working remain poor when elderly – as Silburn (Chapter 9) points out in the context of the United Kingdom: 'The social security system continues to be as much part of the problem as it is part of the solution.'

Or, as has been pointed out elsewhere, poverty remains not despite social security, but because of it (Macarov 1993: 92–101).

The inadequacy of job creation as an anti-poverty strategy

Since the great majority of the very poor are not in the workforce, employment is primarily the solution of choice only for the unemployed poor. It will be immediately recognised that the success of job creation efforts will not improve the lot of the aged and of children, who are out of the workforce (except for children of the unemployed); of the working poor; of single parents whose problem is not being able to work due to small children at home; of farmers; and some other categories of the poor.

The record of national efforts to reduce unemployment substantially is disheartening. Even those countries which have succeeded in somewhat controlling or reducing unemployment have usually done so through the use of part-time, temporary, and/or low-paying jobs, most of which do little to relieve poverty. Because of deliberately narrow definitions and questionable methods of counting, many experts hold that official unemployment figures should always be increased from 50 per cent to 300 per cent. Thus, poverty due to unemployment may be more substantial than generally recognised.

In many countries 'full employment' has become a mantra, constantly repeated, as though reiteration would create facts. Despite years of persistent effort, no country has succeeded in attaining full employment, according to their own definitions, except during wartime. Indeed, it has even been held that the efforts to attain full employment are not only futile, but dangerous to individuals, to the economy and to society (Macarov 1991).

Efforts at deliberately creating jobs, as advocated by Kaseke (Chapter 11), are also not promising. A conference of experts held some time ago to examine the effectiveness of various job creation plans came to the conclusion, in effect, that none of the plans examined created an appreciable number of permanent, full-time jobs (Taggart 1977). Callan and Nolan (Chapter 5) reiterate this finding: permanent job creation, assistance in starting new firms, and temporary job creation 'have very little impact on overall employment or unemployment levels'. It is for this reason that most training and retraining programmes – which, by definition, are designed to prepare people for jobs – do not fulfil their purpose. Even when trainees complete the course, there are few job openings for them, and those that are available are very low-paid. Something similar might be said for plans to widen and deepen educational opportunities. President Johnson is said to have declared, 'We are going to eliminate poverty with education' (quoted in Silver and Silver 1991: 70). The results speak for themselves. Laudable as these activities are in their own right, their success – if achieved – may well be simply a much better educated group of poor people.

The inadequacy of economic development as an anti-poverty strategy

Closely connected to the assumption that full employment will erase much of poverty is reliance on macroeconomic strategies to enhance economic development. This has been phrased by the Irish (Chapter 5) as: 'a rising tide lifts all the boats', meaning that prosperity for the general population trickles down to the poor. Unfortunately, a rising tide may drown those without boats, or create a vicious undertow which does the same thing. Thus, the record of increased overall prosperity as an antidote to poverty is no greater than the other panaceas proposed. As Dirven, Fouarge and Muffels (Chapter 7) note, periods of economic upswings provide no guarantee for solving the issue of poverty. Indeed, relative poverty and deprivation become more serious during periods of economic growth. For example, MacPherson (Chapter 4) notes with respect to Hong Kong that in 1971 the poorest shared 6.2 per cent of all household income, and the richest 49.3 per cent; but by 1991 the share of the poorest had dropped to 4.3 per cent, while that of the richest increased to 52.8 per cent. The same growing inequality has been noted in other countries. In Britain, for example, the poorest tenth of the population saw their real income fall by 6 per cent between 1979 and 1989, while the average rose by 30 per cent and the richest tenth enjoyed a 'staggering' rise of 46 per cent (Oppenheim 1993). Silburn (Chapter 9) found that average income in Britain grew by 33 per cent from 1979 to 1992, while that of the poorest tenth rose by only 9 to 17 per cent. Prosperity, it seems, does not trickle down, but rather bubbles up from the despairing gasps of the poor.

The inadequacies of community and social development as an anti-poverty strategy

Empowering the poor and social development and relevant anti-poverty strategies only work when poverty is conceptualised to embrace a sense of social isolation, alienation, or negative self-images. Such strategies may serve a useful purpose for those involved, but Midgley and Livermore (Chapter 10) call attention to the fact that there have been few systematic attempts to evaluate the effectiveness of community-based anti-poverty programmes. Callan and Nolan (Chapter 5) hold that to expect such programmes to overcome widespread poverty is unrealistic.

The forgotten poor

Mention should be made of two of the largest groups of the poor for whom few programmes seem to have been designed and implemented in the countries reviewed here – the single parent and the working poor.

Single parents

The plight of single parents – usually mothers, and especially those with small children – is usually addressed simply by social assistance programmes. However, even those begun with good intentions and adequate budgets soon fall prey to public disenchantment and government budget cuts. The Aid to Families with Dependent Children (the title has been changed a number of times) programme in the United States was instituted with the image of the white preacher's widow trying to eke out a living for her tow-headed blue-eyed children by giving piano lessons. She was felt to be deserving of help. When the image changed in the public mind to Afro-American unmarried teenaged mothers, the programme rapidly became punitive rather than supportive.

The only other programme undertaken or proposed to help single parents is the provision of child-care facilities so the parent can work. Leaving aside the question of whether public policy is better served by mothers staying at home with their small children, or leaving them in settings which are often overcrowded, under-manned, and unprofessional, the free or subsidised child-care facilities offered or proposed are only for mothers who will go out to work. Those who cannot work or – much more often – cannot find jobs, are not eligible for most such programmes.

The working poor

There is a substantial group of poor people who are in poverty despite the fact that they are working. Midgley and Livermore (Chapter 10) note that in the United States over 40 per cent of the poor aged 16 and over are working regularly. Minimum wage laws are often offered as the solution for this group, but such wages (even when enforced) often leave recipients below the poverty line, especially if they have even moderately large families, since salaries are not based on family structure or need. A full-time worker drawing the minimum wage in the United States will be far below the poverty line if he or she supports a spouse and two children (Macarov 1995: 129). As discussed by Midgley and Livermore (Chapter 10), this problem is addressed in the United States with a tax-rebate programme for low income earners.

Conclusion

Given the myriad groups in poverty and the many programmes designed to help them, directly or indirectly, the current picture is reasonably clear: many people are helped during their poverty, some are helped to leave poverty, but the great majority of the poor in all of the countries reviewed here remain in substantially the same condition. And what of the future?

Cox (Chapter 2) predicts that 'in the future we will witness a significant proportion of the Australian population living in poverty'. Shewell (Chapter 3) argues state efforts to help the needy in Canada have largely been abandoned. MacPherson (Chapter 4) points out that inequality in Hong Kong has grown in recent years. Midgley and Livermore (Chapter 10) hold that the poverty problem in the United States is likely to become even more acute and visible in the future. Silburn (Chapter 9) sees social insecurity and uncertainty becoming more widespread and corrosive in the United Kingdom. Kaseke (Chapter 11) speaks of the reduction of poverty remaining an elusive goal in Zimbabwe. Callan and Nolan (Chapter 5) see a bright future for Irish macroeconomic prospects, but do not venture to indicate how this might translate itself on the poverty front. Tabone (Chapter 6) makes suggestions which he feels might reduce poverty in Malta in the future, as do Gerdes and Pehrson (Chapter 8) in relation to the Philippines, but none of these have yet been acted upon, so their efficacy is open to question. Dirven, Fouarge and Muffels (Chapter 7) speak mainly of the need for further research on the question in the Netherlands.

In summarising the majority view in this volume, it is tempting to conclude that poverty has a rich future (Macarov 1996). It is possible, though, that massive changes in society now being created by rapidly advancing technology will also allow for radical solutions to poverty. For example, Cox (Chapter 2) mentions a 1975 Australian proposal for a guaranteed income for all. This is not a new idea – it was proposed by Thomas More in 1517, and Thomas Paine had the same idea at the end of the eighteenth century. Senator Goldwater proposed such a plan in the United States in 1964, and a modified programme, called the Family Assistance Plan, was narrowly defeated in the United States Congress. The idea has latterly been revived and carried forward by such groups as the Basic Income European Network (de Jager *et al.* 1994), and the Society for the Reduction of Human Labor. The underlying concept is that people should be given enough money to be enabled to lead decent lives without regard for their past, present, or future work.

Although there are ideological and political opponents of the idea of simply giving money to the poor to relieve their condition, the most formidable argument is that it will, as noted by Tabone (Chapter 6), harm incentives to work. Hence the adoption of wage stops in most social security programmes. If, however, technology continues relentlessly to replace human labour, as some contend will invariably happen, the need for some mechanism to support the growing number of people whose work is simply not needed may make the need for some such new societal paradigm inevitable.

Among other possibilities sometimes mentioned is the privatisation of government activities, perhaps through some sort of share-holding by everyone, which would be used to reduce the have/have-not gap. A more fearsome scenario foresees the continued growth of economic inequality leading to social unrest, riots, and revolutionary changes in the socio-economic system. Finally, there is the dystopian view that the poor will not be lifted out of poverty, but that the non-poor will sink into it – a levelling of incomes to be brought about by ecological catastrophes, by political ineptness or manipulation, or by inherent weaknesses in the current production/consumption model. If these dire forecasts are to be averted, it is not enough to keep reinventing the (square) wheels that have failed to eliminate poverty in the past. New, visionary, courageous, convincing models for restructuring society are needed.

REFERENCES

Abramovitz, M. (1993) 'Question: Is the Social Welfare System Inherently Sexist and Racist? Answer: Yes', in Karger, H.J. and Midgley, J. (eds) (1993) *Controversial Issues in Social Policy*, New York: Allyn and Bacon.
de Jager, N.E.M., Graafland, J.J. and Gelauff, G.M.M. (1994) *A Negative Income Tax in a Mini-Welfare State: A Simulation with MIMIC*, The Hague: Central Planbureau.
Dixon, J. (1987) 'Social Security in the Middle East', in Dixon, J. (ed.) *Social Welfare in the Middle East*, London: Croom Helm.
—— (1994) 'Social Security in the Nineties – Challenges and Prospects: Reflections on the Connection between Social Security and Poverty', in *Asia Regional Conference on Social Security (September 14–16 1993), Conference Proceedings*, Hong Kong: Hong Kong Council of Social Services.
—— (1996a) 'Social Security and Poverty Alleviation: Debunking a Myth', in Mok, H. (ed.) *Eradicating Poverty and Employment*, Hong Kong: Hong Kong Social Security Society and Department of Applied Social Studies, Hong Kong Polytechnic University 1996.
—— (1996b) 'Social Security in Transition: An Explorations of Emerging Global Trends', *Proceedings of the 27th International Council on Social Welfare International Conference*, 1, Hong Kong: International Council on Social Welfare.
Gans, H.J. (1967) 'Income Grants and "Dirty Work"', *The Public Interest* 6: 108–22.

Goodwin, L. (1972) *Do the Poor Want to Work? A Social-Psychological Study of Work Orientations*, Washington, DC: Brookings Institution.

Levenberg, M. (1994) 'On the Development of Philanthropic Institutions in Ancient Judaism: Provisions for Poor Travelers', *Nonprofit and Voluntary Section Quarterly* 23 (3): 193–207.

Macarov, D. (1970) *Incentives to Work*, San Francisco: Jossey-Bass.

—— (1980) *Work and Welfare: The Unholy Alliance*, Beverly Hills, CA: Sage.

—— (1991) 'Full Employment is Neither Possible nor Desirable', in Macarov, D. (ed.) *Persisting Unemployment: Can It be Overcome?*, Hull: MCB University Press.

—— (1993) 'Social Security as Poverty's Guardian', *Policy Studies Review* 12 (1/2): 92–101.

—— (1995) *Social Welfare: Structure and Practice*. Thousand Oaks, CA: Sage.

—— (1996) 'Poverty Has a Rich Future', in Didsbury, H.F., Jr. (ed.) *Future Vision: Ideas, Insights, and Strategies*, Bethesda: World Future Society.

Midgley, J. (1993) 'Social Security and Third World Poverty: The Challenges to Policymakers', *Policy Studies Review* 12 (1/2): 133–43.

Oppenheim, C. (1993) *Poverty: The Facts*, London: Child Poverty Action Group.

Room, G. (1993) *Anti-Poverty Action-Research in Europe*, Bristol: SAUS Press.

Roper, R.H. (1991) *Persistent Poverty: The American Dream Turned Nightmare*, New York: Plenum.

Ryan, W. (1974) 'Blaming the Victim: Ideology Serves the Establishment', in Ryan, W. (ed.) *The Poverty Establishment*, Englewood Cliffs, NJ: Prentice Hall.

Silver, H. and Silver, P. (1991) *An Educational War on Poverty: American and British Policy-Making: 1960–1980*, Cambridge, MA: Cambridge University Press.

Taggart, R. (ed.) (1977) *Job Creation: What Works?*, Salt Lake City, Utah: Olympus.

United Nations (1995) *Poverty*, New York: United Nations.

Index